Coraggio!

Lessons for Living From an Italian Grandmother Despite Illness, Pain and Loss

By
Lisa K. Gigliotti, J.D.

With Courage,
you can!

Coraggio!

Lisa Gigliotti

Table of Contents

Introduction   vii

Lezione Uno: Coraggio, Leeza (Lesson One: Courage, Lisa)
**   The Importance of Courage   1**

Chapter 1   A Nursing Home Deposit   3
Chapter 2   Invasion of the Bone Tormentors   8
Chapter 3   *"Coraggio, Leeza. Coraggio."* (Courage, Lisa.
                Courage.)   17
Chapter 4   Old World Life Lessons in Courage for
                Nonna   24
Chapter 5   This Can't Be Happening to Me!   39
Chapter 6   The Accident   47
Chapter 7   Neurotransmitter Imposters   59
Chapter 8   In the Depths of the Soul's Dark Night   81

Table of Contents

Chapter 9   Life Lessons About Courage from Nonna   94

Chapter 10   Willow Branches   113

**Lezione Due: Il Malocchio (Lesson Two: The Evil Eye)
The Courage to Take Charge of the Aspects
of Life You *Can* Control   117**

Chapter 11   The Evil Eye   119

Chapter 12   Grab Courage, Take Charge!   126

Chapter 13   Take Charge of the Aspects of Health Care Within Your Control   131

Chapter 14   Take Charge of Your Health: Find a Doctor Who Will Work With You   138

Chapter 15   Take Charge of Your Health: Educate Yourself About Treatment Options   148

Chapter 16   Take Charge of Your Attitude   157

Chapter 17   Take Charge of Thoughts and Actions Through Reframing   162

Chapter 18   Take Charge of the Aspects of Your Destiny that You Can Control   167

Chapter 19   From *"Mangia tutti!"* to *"Mangia bene!"*   172

Chapter 20   Take Charge of Your Diet   181

Chapter 21   Lifestyle is a Choice Over Which You Have Control   186

Chapter 22   Take Charge of Your Health: Exercise, Body Weight and Muscle Tone   192

Chapter 23   Focus on the Positive to Accomplish Lifestyle Change   201

Chapter 24   *Buona Notte*! Take Charge of the Aspects of Sleep that You Can Control   205

Chapter 25   Take Charge of Non-Traditional Healing Opportunities   208

Chapter 26   Deal With What I am Able and *"Ciao"* ... Let Go of the Rest   213

Table of Contents

Chapter 27 Denial as a Means of Control   218

Chapter 28 Caution Against Controlling Others as a Means of Control   220

Chapter 29 Taking Charge of Grief   225

Lezione Tre: Amore (Lesson Three: Love)
The Courage to Love Yourself When You Feel Unlovable;
The Courage to Love Another Despite Being Hurt;
The Courage to Feel Love Again After the Loss
of One You Love   231

Chapter 30 The Big Italian Family Fight   233

Chapter 31 Self-Love   238

Chapter 32 The Importance of Positive Attitude in Achieving Self-Love, Less Pain and Life Gusto   243

Chapter 33 The Importance of Cleaning Out Emotional Baggage to Clear the Path to Loving Yourself   253

Chapter 34 Importance of Reducing Fear to Increase Love   257

Chapter 35 The Importance of Humor in Loving Yourself   266

Chapter 36 The Importance of Life Purpose as a Key Component of Self-Love   270

Chapter 37 Understanding Processed Food Cravings to Achieve Self-Loving Food Choices   282

Chapter 38 Family Love and Tradition to Achieve Lifestyle Balance   285

Chapter 39 Loving Others   289

Chapter 40 Love From Others   291

Chapter 41 Love From Others at the Time of Loss   297

Chapter 42 The Importance of Giving Love to a Caregiver   300

Table of Contents

Chapter 43   That's Amore. Dating When You Look Disabled
or "Different"   309

Chapter 44   The Marriage Relationship and Chronic
Illness   314

Chapter 45   Remembering to Love Yourself When Others are
not Loving Toward You   317

Chapter 46   The Courage to Love Yourself   325

Epilogue   331
Bibliography   333

Introduction

As a teenager I could never have imagined or been prepared for the ugly blows that struck against what should have been the remaining few years of youthful lightheartedness. With rapid-fire succession came a crippling disease so ferocious it quickly forced me into a wheelchair, a life-threatening onset of a little-known neuromuscular disease, a tragic auto accident which ripped away the lives of my mother and grandmother, and the culmination of tragedies thwarting medical school plans. By age twenty-five, I was alone, in a wheelchair, and grappling to deal with two chronic illnesses, constant physical pain, and the devastating loss of my beloved caregivers and life goals.

To whom could I turn for my daily personal care and companionship? Where would I find strength and wisdom to battle the relentless illnesses and engulfing grief? I readily and most

humbly admitted that I was no superhero. It was not noble heroism or extraordinary talent that enabled me to surpass barriers
of physical disability and immobilizing grief. My fortune was the
indelible example of four strong women.

This book is dedicated to my Italian Grandmother (Nonna)
Saveria Rizzo Gigliotti, to Great-Grandmother Giuseppina Rizzo,
to Mom, Julia Barczay-Gigliotti and to Hungarian Grandmother
(Nagymama) Anna Barczay. The stoic lives these four stalwart
women led and the stories they told were invaluable lessons
about love, and faith, and courage. Each maternal figure exhibited extraordinary faith and unwavering courage to overcome
unfathomable trials; all done with grace to accept what was not
possible to change, with hope for a better life and the determination to work toward it; and with refusal to dwell as victim, but
rather with positive focus toward serving others. Little did they
know that they modeled for me the very vital elements of what I
would need to overcome the challenges of my young life.

Nagymama tucked her beautiful, curly-blond, six year-old
Julia under her right arm and her eight-year-old Anna under her
left arm, and attempted to usher them through the hate-filled
and murder-ridden cities of Europe in war-savaged 1945. Her
courage and faith achieved safe passage to America for her, her
husband and daughters. Nagymama held her regal head high as,
accustomed to a former life of royal wealth and servants; she instead cleaned the affluent houses of Grosse Pointe, Michigan elite
or labored in the humble laundry department of Detroit's Henry
Ford Hospital.

Great-Grandmother Giuseppina, incapacitated by seasickness, bundled her eight-year-old, five year-old, and ten-month-
old children in the steerage-class berth of a lice-infested and
storm-tossed ocean liner. Penniless, uneducated and without
knowledge of English, her courage and faith achieved safe passage to America in hopes of a better life for her husband and
daughters.

And to my sweet, but fiercely determined Nonna, whose courage is the centerpiece of this book, it was her voice of encouragement I heard in the back of my young mind during its most agonizing moment: "*Coraggio, Leeza, Coraggio.*" This simple woman, with only a seventh grade education bore examples of courage which served as lessons on living life with *gusto* despite chronic illness, nagging pain and devastating loss.

What does courage have to do with chronic illness, pain, grief, love, lifestyle, or faith? Courage is at the foundation of every tool for handling adversity in life. Adversity will always be present, but what your life will be depends on what you do with adversity. Will you begrudge adversity and spend each day in negativity and limitation? Will you fall victim to adversity and spend each day in helplessness, self-pity or excuses? Will you find joy, gratitude and laughter, live life with *amore* and *gusto*, despite adversity? Will you find purpose or a desire to change as a consequence of adversity? Will you discover spiritual meaning behind adversity?

The series of *Coraggio* books are intended to share Nonna's lessons for living. Nonna's *Lezioni Uno—Sette* (Lessons One—Seven) are grouped into four books. This book, *Lezioni Uno—Tre* (Lessons One—Three) shows how to call on *coraggio* (courage) for the fortitude to take charge of your life and for the strength to shape your life to its fulfilling purpose.

It was inspiring for me to read about medical missionaries while I was bed-ridden and it was encouraging for me to gain insight through spiritual or inspirational books during other difficult periods in my life. Yet it was a physical struggle to hold a book open and upright. The constant fight against a bookbinding's desire to slam closed caused added pain to my sore elbows, throbbing shoulders and pinching neck. The weight of the book often won out over arm muscles fatigued by myasthenia gravis. I promised myself when *Coraggio* was published I would make it ergonomically friendly regardless of the expense. All the readers with aching elbows, throbbing shoulders, pinched necks, muscle weakness, one hand or no hands will be able to have at it. *Coraggio* was designed to have a light cover and a spiral binding that will lay flat and remain open. The design should enable a person with arthritis, neuromuscular challenges or missing limbs to prop the book at eye level and let go until it is time to turn a page.

Coraggio's format is structured for the person with low stamina, diminished focus or a hectic life. The chapters are short and the headings are descriptive. If you are running short on energy or time you will be able to zero in on your interest or need by referring to the Table of Contents. *Lezione Uno* (Lesson One) is the story of how Nonna learned courage and about the symptoms that led to my diagnoses of rheumatoid arthritis and myasthenia gravis. I am not offended if your greater interest is in self-help tips for taking charge, wherein if you choose to, you can skip the first section and land in the many "take charge" chapters. This book is written for *You!*

Each chapter is summarized with at least one Courage Keeper—a message to take with you, to reflect on and to encourage you when needed. Courage Keeper is a play on the word "keeper", meaning to take with you, but with a second meaning intended to remind you that you are the keeper of your own courage. You alone possess the ability to pull forth the courage within you to face and charge through whatever is facing you at that moment. The Courage Keeper end-of-chapter bullets were also designed to facilitate speed-readers or for an easy refresher.

My life has been immeasurably blessed by friends and family who brought richness and joy. Heartfelt gratitude for Cheryl, Kathy and David, who read unending *Coraggio* drafts and provided edits. And for Maura who, despite her own December 23rd love-of-her-life loss, was unceasing in the mantra, "... this book *must* be published!"

Lezione Uno: Coraggio, Leeza
(Lesson One: Courage, Lisa)

The Importance of Courage

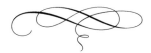

CHAPTER 1

A Nursing Home Deposit

Splashes of blues and grays whisked before my lowered eyes. The drab color of nursing home corridor carpet was interrupted by splotches of stains; spills as dinner trays collected from disinterested recipients were carried to their designated slot in the stainless steel cart parked in the hallway. Or perhaps the amorphous blotches, now discolored, were the result of bodily fluids best left unimagined.

The young nurse aide had already reached a brisk pace. She was tiny; I was amazed that by mid-length of the hallway she could reach such velocity, pushing both me and my wheelchair against the drag of carpet, not that I weighed much more than a hundred pounds myself. Since the onset of the muscle weakening disease myasthenia gravis merely weeks ago I had lost the ability to chew and swallow, and with it had lost body weight.

Fifteen minutes earlier I had arrived at the nursing home via a medical transport van. The driver of the van had backed my wheelchair down the van's ramp and deposited me in the nursing facility foyer. I waited, hunched over with exhaustion as staff fussed to determine which nurse aide I was assigned to that evening. She who was to have the honor was beckoned via intercom. I had always lacked patience. It was doubly frustrating for me to be dependent on another person to push my manual wheelchair, especially if I had to wait for help. *I wonder how long it will be until she arrives. It would only take me seconds to get to my room if I could just walk on my own two feet!* But today I did not care how long I had to wait; I was too spent to care.

Mercifully the nurse arrived in fairly short time and dutifully navigated me to the last room on the right-hand side of the nursing facility's east wing. As we sped through hallways we passed other residents in their wheelchairs, old shrunken bodies parked in the hall for the afternoon. Some stared straight ahead, bulged-eyes glazed and mouths agape, without noticing me. Others called out to me in their dementia as we whisked past. I responded to none. I was not ashamed that I could not extend even a tiny bit of human kindness—a nod, a smile, some acknowledgement of their presence. Still hunched in my wheelchair, I preferred to fix my gaze on the soiled carpet rolling by beneath the footrests until we reached my room.

I was impressed by the strength of the diminutive nurse aide. Locking the brakes of the wheelchair after parking it alongside my hospital bed she wrapped her arms in a bear hug around me. Gently she hoisted me in a seated position from the wheelchair, pivoting slightly until my bottom was planted solidly on the bed. *Ohhhh ... relief.* As I lay back she helped lift and swing my legs into a lying position on the bed. I lay there, eyes closed, body fully extended, grateful for what seemed an extreme luxury, but without an ounce of energy to move or speak.

The young aide was intuitive and sensitive. Without prompts she pulled the ultra-bleached sheets over me so that I would not have to use my bandaged, bruised and sore arms. Perhaps she had noticed the bulging pressure bandages surrounding the insertion sites on both arms from the large, rigid dialysis needles that had been in place for hours. I felt cold and weak after the day-long blood dialysis at the nearby hospital. That was the only reason I was glad to be back in bed and covered with a sheet.

I glanced toward my roommate; a compulsion to look similar to the attraction that draws eyes to the gruesome scene of an accident. It used to frighten me to catch her locked gaze burning directly into my eyes. But in its intensity was a rather odd, dark void born of an absence of cognition.

Our beds were a mere four feet apart. While the staff caringly administered to her tube feedings, medications or sponge baths they spoke in hushed tones to me. They also compassionately spoke to her in loud tones, impossible for me to ignore.

I gathered glimpses of her former life from various nurses and aides. Until recently, she had been a striking, energetic mother of two young children, her knockout figure due in part to having been an aerobics instructor. She was married to a wealthy doctor, their family home in Beverly Hills, California.

How could this be? She had two perfect children, one boy and one girl. She had the perfect husband who was a fine-looking doctor. *And what neighborhood in the world could be more perfect than Beverly Hills?* I could not shake the perplexing irony of the present contracted, semi-comatose woman to the perfect face, perfect body, perfect husband, perfect family, perfect home, and perfect life story.

Over numerous days I pieced together the episode that added the ironic but cruelly wicked twist to this perfect life story. This gorgeous, athletic mother and her attractive doctor-husband were on an extravagant vacation in Mexico, on an exotic scuba dive leagues deep in the warm Pacific Ocean waters. The air hose leading from her oxygen tank to her mouth became entangled in seaweed. She was separated from her only source of life-giving oxygen with a world of nothing but suffocating water overpowering her. By the time they got her to the surface of the ocean she was unconscious and no longer breathing. They hoisted her drowned, lifeless body onto the dive boat.

Her doctor-husband performed the most heroic and intense emergency resuscitative treatment of his life. He succeeded in reviving his precious wife, wherein her heart restarted its pulsating and he maintained the strenuous forcing of his frantic breath into her lungs for what seemed hours. But her brain had been without oxygen for longer than it could tolerate. In that mysterious crossroads between no oxygen long enough for significant damage but short enough to cheat death, the revived and revered wife remained in a persistent, semi-conscious state.

Can she see me in some dim, blurry corner of her damaged but importunate mind? Today her intense, wide-eyed stare did not startle me as much as in the days prior. Instead I felt great compassion for this beautiful soul. She was only in her 30s.

I turned away my face toward the door and pretended I was asleep when on Sundays her little girl and boy would be handled by their father to their mother's bedside. I wanted to provide some shred of privacy in this intrusive, cramped and unwelcoming nursing home environment. Their eyes remained on the tile floor, their voices silent. Their father spoke for them as a loving, devoted husband. The pall of broken hearts was palpable in the sterile, insensitive room. My own heart strained to the point of bursting as a mere unwilling participant in this incomprehensibly tragic scene. The compassion stirred within me not only out of empathy for all four members of this devastated family, but because I believed I would become well enough to leave this forsaken place for my tiny, comforting apartment with a phone over which I could hear voices of loved ones and speak a cogent thought.

I was not so sure about the prospect of my roommate or the other parked elderly residents I passed in the hall.

Use courage to:

- In times of desperation, realize you have power within.

Chapter 2

Invasion of the Bone Tormentors

I COULD NOT BELIEVE I REALLY WAS HERE, IN THIS PLACE OF INTERMINGLED odors of urine and disinfectant.

"Dear GOD ... I am only twenty-five years old! Wasn't it only a couple of years ago that I was preparing for medical school? Back then I attended pre-med classes in the red-bricked Albertus Magnus Science Hall at Aquinas College. In the evenings I pulled on jeans under the white nurse dress so I could pedal my bike to my nurse aide night shift job. Aquinata Hall, for lack of a more suitable description, was an assisted living

and nursing home for retired Grand Rapid Dominican Sisters, those beautiful servants of God, who in the spirit of the Italian Saint Dominic had spent their entire lives selflessly working to help others. Now in their years of infirmity or dementia, they needed care as they faced transition to the new and glorious life they believed would follow. Aquinata Hall was more than a nursing facility; it was a community in which a life of prayer and faith continued. I was privileged to work in that community, helping to bathe, feed, and change clothes and bedding for those sweet nuns.

Ever hear of Southern Italian stubbornness called *testadura* (hard-headedness) or Hungarian Bull's Blood (*Egri Bekaver*) wine? Well, I studied, played and worked with all the determination of *testdadura* and with all the strength of Hungarian bull's blood. Add with it a Catholic upbringing steeped in social justice, and no matter how tired I was, how gruesome the bedsore or how combative the dementia, I made it to work and administered care with a smile, joke or soothing words. That was the Lisa spirit I knew and expected of myself. *Keep driving yourself toward your goals. Treat every person with dignity and kindness.*

Now, only a few years forward, what had happened to the goal of a career extending compassionate medical care to others? *Instead, <u>you</u> are a nursing home patient. Compassion? Toward your fellow residents you are averse to extending the basic human kindness of eye contact, nod or "hi."*

I used to love to run. I ran one to three miles everyday, sprinting off stress after college classes or concluding my day with a delighted dash through impressive tree-lined, lamp lit East Grand Rapids neighborhood streets.

God, You know I loved to run. God, <u>You</u> were the one who formed me with smarts to exceed in the hard sciences. It was <u>You</u> who instilled in me a heart that acutely cared about helping others. <u>You</u> were the one who gave me the strength to work as a nurse aide evenings and weekends through those full-time college years. Why God, did you take *that from me? Why God did you bring me to this place where I am now the one dependent on nurse aides?*

In my bleached-sheet bed and fluorescent lit, smelly room, far from the peaceful, stately, golden-leafed, tree-lined streets of East Grand Rapids, I feverishly demanded answers from an all-knowing sovereign. Hearing no heavenly response, I ended my conversation with God. With feelings of confusion, frustration, abandonment and isolation I turned to the only person I felt was left: me. *How did I ever get here?*

My thoughts scurried back through time to the life-turning event of only five years past. Home from college for the summer, I had made an appointment to see the family doctor. Holding out both hands, I showed him the grossly swollen and angry red knuckles. Using both of his hands, he palpated over each of the knuckle joints of my hands.

He felt for inflammatory warmth and then pressed down gingerly. "Does it hurt when I press down on your joint?"

"No, not really. It is sore when you press down, but it is not painful."

I felt foolish that I had sought his attention, yet upon his examination was merely sore. He had already chastised me for being several pounds overweight. I decided it was the time to admit to myself the symptoms that had scared me into making the appointment. It was also time to confess what I had been hiding from everyone but Dad and *Nonna,* Italian for grandmother, by which we affectionately called her.

"I started having intense, jabbing pain, deep in my bones, especially at night. Oh, and I keep dropping things. I know it sounds weird, but I don't drop only heavy things; small things too. It is as if they slip right through my fingers."

The doctor did not respond to my comment, but remained silent, entirely focused as he used two fingers from each hand to completely encircle each joint; pressing for bogginess, feeling for warmth. After he finished with one joint he turned to the preprinted examination notes sheet, circled the corresponding finger on the anatomical diagram, and wrote an undecipherable note. I squinted my best to try and read next to the circle. Without any eye contact or remark he turned back to my hand and moved to the next joint. I decided against speaking, not wanting to disturb his concentration.

He finished squeezing the last finger and broke the prolonged silence. "I would like to take a look at your knees."

I slid back on the exam table until my legs were extended and hiked the exam gown above my knees. Using the back of his hand against my skin, he slowly moved from my shin up toward the knee, feeling for an increase in warmth that signified tissue inflammation.

"Your knee joints are also warm and inflamed. Do they hurt?"

"Yes. I didn't mention it to you earlier because I thought the hurt might be due to the weight I gained last semester." I was embarrassed. The truth was I blamed a lot of the swelling and soreness throughout my body on the fact that I had gained weight.

The doctor turned back to his notes, flipped to the opposite side of the sheet and jotted. He pulled out another sheet whose preprint resembled a checklist and began making marks in the boxes of the left margin. He finally turned back to me, crossed his arms, and sighed. "From the symptoms you described and from my physical examination of your hands and other joints, you could have a disease we call rheumatoid arthritis. The symptoms could indicate an even more serious problem: bone cancer. I don't think it is bone cancer but I want to rule out any possibility. I want my nurse to get some blood from you today so we can run some tests. We should have the test results within a week. So before you leave today make an appointment to come back and talk to me." He turned to leave but stopped at the door, looking at the floor as he hesitated in thought. "Do you want me to call your father to talk to him about what we discussed?"

It was 1981, before medical record confidentiality laws. I was twenty years old, sprung from the ledge of legal minority, leaping into adulthood. Yet, he could have called my father and discussed any of my private health information without the current-day legal repercussions. *See, the doc still considered me a kid; or at least he isn't sure.*

"No thanks. I understand everything you said and I can relate it to my father."

I went to a small room at the end of the hall and his nurse took several vials of blood from my arm. We made light conversation so as to avoid discussing the possibility of what would be revealed from the dark garnet liquid she was extracting. I made arrangements with the overly sympathetic lady at the reception counter to come back a week later.

Tell a young drama queen she might have bone cancer and let her wait a week. It was all too easy at that age to let my mind drift to fatalism. I had not really told anyone except the doctor, but for the past couple of weeks the deep bone pain was so viciously hot and stabbing that I thought the possibility of bone cancer was not too far fetched.

Limbo week grew unbearably long. I engaged my mind elsewhere, actually applying full faculties and focus to studying for my summer calculus class weekly exam. The industrious focus served more purpose than mere distraction as I achieved a perfect score on the exam and received the highest score in the class for the third week in a row.

I had spent the first part of the year in a small town north of Galway, Ireland. Aquinas College, where I spent the first two years of undergrad had an Irish study abroad program. The second semester of every academic year, Aquinas College rented several holiday cottages close to the sea, sent along two professors and let about two dozen students roam the Irish country where classes were held three nights a week in one of the thatched-roof cottages. We were fortunate in that our imported professors were Professor Betty, an ironic mix of outspoken irreverence and wit beset with impeccable etiquette, and Sister Mona, a calming mother figure with poetic grace. Most of our classes were held seated on the stone floor of their cottage, the smell and warmth of peat fire behind us.

Toward the middle of the semester, my feet began to hurt a few hours after I ran. If I had been honest with myself I would have admitted that my feet also hurt before I ran and ached when I was not running. While the weather was cold and rainy most days, it was not as harsh as the cold Michigan winter. I loved to run in the Irish drizzle, looking out through the grey mist onto the contrasting richly emerald green hillsides, their lushness interrupted by grey, craggy rocks. *Aye ... a Harsh Beauty she is.* As we were in the rural west of Ireland, I could run for an hour without seeing another human or hearing a car, phone or stereo. Just the soul-nourishing sound of stillness, the crashing ocean, the wind rushing across the bog, or the "bahhh" of sheep on a velvety green hillside.

I began to make excuses for the reason my feet ached. *Your feet ache because they are constantly cold and wet. It might not be the bitter cold of Michigan winter, but it is that damp cold that chills to the core; or it is your own fault your feet hurt because most likely you have fallen arches; after all you've gained at least ten pounds from drinking Guinness and eating locally churned, butter-laden, Irish brown soda bread since landing on this ol' sod.*

Our small town of Tully Cross consisted of one church, two tiny stores and two pubs. I could always find a classmate to accompany me to one of the two pubs across the street each evening. A music lover to the core of my being, nothing tickled my heart better than listening to the town folk who came along to the pub, instrument in hand. I could not imagine a better Nirvana than to sit, sipping on a pint of creamy Guinness fresh from a motherland tap, while Johnny sat a table in the corner, put his fiddle to his chin and started with an Irish reel. Paddy would show up fifteen minutes later to keep beat with his bodhran, an Irish drum consisting of a tight skin stretched over a wood circular rim, held in one hand and beaten with both ends of a drumstick. Sean came along with a tin whistle to liven the already peppy jig. But my favorite was to hear the Irish ballads. I learned more of the tormented, oppressive Irish history from listening to these emotional Irish ballads than from Sister Mona's Irish History class.

I sat, nodding my head and tapping my toe to the beat, joining my voice to the patriotic ballads, and sipping Guinness, draining every last drop from the pint glass. I never dreamed the thick and smooth nectar was adding another 200 calories per pint to my daily calorie count. Oh sure, it was easy to convince myself the nagging, throbbing in my feet was related to weight gain.

The upstairs of our whitewashed thatched-roof Irish cottage was one open room shared by Pegeen, Marilyn and me. It was a months-long pajama party of shared discovery, homesickness, future dreams, laughter and tears. It was also a Petri dish of shared germs. Pegeen succumbed to a fearsome cold shortly after we arrived. As she began to mend, the ruthless virus took over my body. Marilyn was next. None of us three escaped the virus' brutality.

Fever, congestion, coughing fits might have been mitigated with Vitamin C, herbal tea or medication, but none of the U.S. natural remedies or pharmaceuticals to which we were accustomed for healing were readily available. There were at least twenty-four hours where I laid helpless to bouts of body-shaking chills contrasted with a sweat-soaked fever-induced flu-like ache that seemed to accompany virulent viruses that beset my joints. For days after the fever abated I noticed that the knuckles on my hand were enlarged with hot redness and swelling. I had to wrestle with my onyx-stoned Dominican High School Class of 1979 ring in order to force it free over the swollen middle joint of my ring finger. *Your ring is tight because you've put on some hefty pounds, girl. What did you expect, Miss Chubby? And residual from the viral flu could be adding to the swelling and soreness.* It was all too logical. My analytical mind attributed the red swollen joints to the after-effects of a nasty virus, or the incessant chilling damp, or the weight gain and laxing of prior fanatical exercise. There was nothing more notable, so I blew off any further serious thought.

The spellbinding Irish study abroad concluded. Ever so reluctantly I left the beauty and soul-solace of the emerald isle I had come to love and returned to my father's home in Michigan for the summer. *At least it will be warmer in Michigan,* I thought. I signed up for a calculus class at the local community college and luckily landed a summer job in the school library.

Then, suddenly and fiercely, it hit. I woke in the middle of the night locked into a fetal position. None of my joints would unhinge from the mysterious, evil, stranglehold. The pain was excruciating, originating like a fiery hot poker at the core of my bones. *OOWWwww!* I could hear the scream of agony in my mind as I was shaken awake by pain. *Don't scream out loud! You'll awaken and frighten everyone in the house!* I turned a stiffened neck slightly so my mouth was stuffed into the pillow and uttered an almost silent, muffled scream, panting through the shockwaves of merciless pain.

At dinnertime, the following day, I shuffled stiffly from the kitchen counter to the dining table. The dinner plate suddenly slipped through my hands. It landed on the floor, facedown, with a clatter and splatter of food. Had an unforeseen demon force flipped the plate up and then cruelly slammed it face down on to the floor? I was sleep-deprived with an under layer of unrecognized fear. The sight of food splattered across my slippers and floor and the thought of having to exert joint movement to clean it and prepare another dinner seemed exasperating. *Don't cry; it will waste too much energy.*

The middle of that night was again spent in screaming-out-loud, throbbing, locked joints. When the family doctor's office opened in the morning I called, made an appointment, received the doctor's speculative diagnoses, and had blood taken for testing. I was left to a week of limbo until the test results were returned and translated to me by the doctor.

The day after the preliminary doctor appointment, a limp now added to my stiff shuffled gait and I dragged myself to a backyard vinyl-strapped lounge chair. There could be nothing better to take my mind from the horrific potential diseases listed by the doctor than to bake my winter white skin in the Midwest summer sun. The solar heat dulled the relentless ache in all my joints. I let my other senses soak in the goodness as well—the majesty of the spade-leaved, 50-foot poplar tree in our backyard, the excited chatter of varied species of birds as they criss-crossed above. But as soon as I closed my eyes and lay my head back on the vinyl-strapped chaise lounge, worried thoughts tried to take over.

I pulled out *The Trinity*, an epic tale of Irish love and tragedy, written by Leon Uris. With my recent Irish experiences I found it very easy to become thoroughly immersed into the unstoppable and fearless, humorous Irish character and harsh beauty of Ireland's landscape. And so limbo week passed.

Use courage to:
- In the face of potential yet unknown peril, realize you have control over feelings of anxiety or hopelessness.
- In the face of potential yet unknown peril, find a means of diverting your thoughts into positive affirmation or soul-soothing play.

CHAPTER 3

"Coraggio, Leeza. Coraggio." (Courage, Lisa. Courage.)

THERE I WAS, ONE WEEK LATER, WITH THIS SMALL-STATURE DOCTOR WHO held the large truth about my fate.

I considered myself a tough twenty-year-old. From fourteen years old, I had helped my father raise my two brothers and sister and me. On the positive side of weekly meal planning, shopping, cooking, laundry, phone call inquiries from a young age, I had become independent earlier than most of my peers.

Until that moment in the doctor's office awaiting the results of my blood tests, it had never occurred to me to ask someone to accompany me at the follow-up appointment. I was alone. *Besides, Dad is working the afternoon shift just now. Mom lives in California.* I reasoned with myself that it was logical to be here unaccompanied. I was accustomed to flying solo into difficult situations and resolving them to the best of my adolescent ability. I did not feel sorry for myself or feel scared. *You are an adult now. You can handle whatever news is about to come your way. Welcome to adulthood, sister.*

I would not have known there was anything seriously wrong by the matter-of-fact demeanor with which the doctor entered the room. He pulled the wheeled stool close to the exam table where I sat on the edge, legs dangling. "The test results were conclusive for rheumatoid arthritis."

Okay, well at least it's not bone cancer.

"I was alarmed to see your sedimentation rate was very high. We use your sedimentation rate to calibrate the activity of the disease. A high sedimentation rate such as yours is an indication that your disease is very active; acute; serious.

That did not sound very good. "Well, I guess I should not be surprised I had something going on by the intense level of pain. What treatment is recommended for a cure?"

"There is no cure for rheumatoid arthritis." His voice was firm. Without barely a pause he finished. "It is a chronic, auto-immune disease."

What's he talking about no cure? This is the 1980s. They are making medical breakthrough discoveries everyday for life-threatening diseases. This is just arthritis! How hard can that be to figure out? This guy doesn't understand. I have a future. I am going to be a doctor and I have the drive and God-given heart and mind to be a doctor.

I inquired in my best twenty-year-old businesslike tone, "I understand. Just tell me what I have to do so I can get back to college this Fall. I am pre-med and I need to continue my classes and start studying for the medical college entrance exam."

"I don't think you *do* understand, dear." He stopped and sighed. He appeared to be struggling to find how and what to say next. His pause was interminable. "This rheumatoid arthritis, it is a serious debilitating disease." His speech took on a patronizing tone. "Your blood tests show you have a severe case. It *will* cripple you. You will not be able to finish school."

I was incredulous at his damning prognosticative statement. *How dare he tell me I will not be able to finish what I started, to reach a goal I have been thus far successful working toward. Every statement uttered from his mouth is totally damning. He has not presented any treatment options or hope for a best-case scenario.*

He saw the look of disdain on my face and quickly tried to repair the situation. "But don't worry, dear. They have nice homes for you to live in. The homes are all set up to take care of you there."

He dangled this last sentence out there so dripping with fake sweetness it sickened me. He had a slight smile on his face. *Unbelievable. He is smiling. Is your smile supposed to be comforting? How in the world do you know whether I will be crippled, much less crippled to the point where I will need total care in a nursing home? Do you know more than you are telling me? And why did you just tell me that I would not finish school? Don't you know I am not like those other college students who end up taking time off from school or joining the Peace Corps to figure out what they want to do with their life?*

I had known from the time I was a little girl that I wanted to be a doctor. Becoming a doctor was in my blood and in my spirit. My childhood was spent building block upon building block, reaching closer to the goal. I would lie awake at night formulating theories in my mind about what type of salve or poultice would heal my cat. After falling asleep I would dream of mixing together ingredients that produced a miraculous cure. Upon awakening I would mix the dream-revealed ingredients and administer them to the cat while stroking her and whispering reassuring words. No dreams of ponies or bubbles for this little girl. I spent hours inventing and constructing health-related devices. As far back as grade school I had read books filled with science, mystery and medicine. I had been born with an unquenchable curiosity for science, a heart filled with compassion and a desire to nurture. With all of my soul I knew I would be a healer. My determination seemed unstoppable.

But here at twenty years old, closer to the physician goal than ever, I found myself with this supposed man of medicine who had just told me I would be dependent on others instead of healing others. *Doesn't he know I am a jock with a body built and trained like an ox?* I was not a cutesy, petite teen gymnast or a tall twiggish high-school basketball player. I had a chunky adolescent physique that I turned into sheer force during flag football games in high school and college. I had never been sleek or coordinated enough to be one of the better members of the track team, so I ran the distance events and used my body mass to thrust the shot put and discus. I ran one to three miles everyday of my life through all of Michigan's four seasons. There was nothing more splendid, more soul-filling than running under the bright gold and orange-leaved fall trees. Fully emblazoned color surrounded me and shin-deep, crispy, musty brown leaves crunched beneath my running shoes, filling my nostrils and ears. A few months later that same run was a delicate dance through several inches of fresh powder snow, thousands of diamonds sparkling off the streetlights in the dark of winter mornings and evenings.

Doesn't he know I am a young person filled with dreams and energetic enthusiasm? How could anyone tell a young person they cannot achieve their goal, to abandon their dreams? Doesn't he know I am born of Calabrese testadura (hard-head) stock?

My Italian grandparents on my father's side were stubborn and courageous enough to start a new life at a young age, on a new continent where no one spoke their language. My mother and her parents had been courageous and clever enough to leave their Hungarian estate, escape through a World War II-torn Europe to the deep South of the United States, for heaven's sake! I was raised hearing stories from both sets of grandparents, seeing before me living examples of courage; determined effort to never give up dreams and that hope always existed. My genes are embedded with stubbornness and courage. *How can this one diminutive man banish to hell all my grand dreams and all my hopes with it? Doesn't he know to whom he is talking?*

I am sure my fists were gripped at my side and my jaw set in fighting-for-life mode.

He did not seem to notice and continued his post-diagnosis discourse. "Start taking eight aspirin a day. Take up to twenty a day if your joints still hurt or continue to be swollen. If the aspirin doesn't help you will need to see a specialist. Make an appointment to see me in four weeks ..."

I drove to Nonna's directly from the doctor's office. The drive was only two miles down Harper Avenue, a main thoroughfare through the city of Saint Clair Shores. Nonna was the only maternal figure for me in Michigan now that my mother and her mother (*Nagymama*) lived in California. I pulled up in front of Nonna's red-brick ranch, one of the many small tract homes leading a half block to Lake Saint Clair. She was sitting on the raised cement porch, trying to catch a lake breeze through the heat and heavy humidity. I knew of no relative whose home had central air conditioning in the summer of 1981.

I could see her smile when I got out of the car. Nonna always smiled when she saw me. Stiffly, I climbed one-by-one the three cement porch steps and stood in front of her.

"It was not good news," I calmly informed her.

"Let's go inside, Leeza." She spoke in the reassuring Nonna tone.

The spell of her calm positive tone brought a sense of comfort to me in this critical moment. Seated in the wrought iron front porch settee she hooked her arm through my elbow so I could retrieve her from the sunken, burnt-orange, brown and yellow floral vinyl cushions and escort her into the house. The swelter of heat and humidity took away my breath as we went inside.

It was stifling in her tiny front room, but not as suffocating as the reality I was about to acknowledge to her. I told her what the doctor had told me, that the disease was permanent and debilitating.

"I told him I was studying to be a doctor." I said with righteous tone. "And he told me, 'No, the disease will cripple you." I started to stumble with my words. Weakness was not allowed in our proud *Calabrese* world. I took a deep breath to steady myself then rushed on.

"He told me I would be crippled, but not to worry because they have nice institutions where people can take care of me for the rest of my life! Nonna, the doctor was totally thoughtless, really insensitive. He was … he was a …"

I wanted to call the doctor a swear word. I used swear words since I was in high school, even though many of my Catholic school friends did not. I had the perfect swear word at the front of my tongue to call the doctor. Nonna would excuse me for swearing, given the circumstances. But I thought I better not. I was raised to respect adults, my grandparents especially, and I did not want to pile any stress on Nonna to the already hefty news.

"He was a … jerk!"

Nonna did not say anything. She did not interrupt me. There was no embracing as our family was not demonstrative of affection in the years after my mother had left our family. There was no crying. Crying was emotional, not practical and not the strong *Calabrese* way.

We sat there in silence, the fan in the kitchen window and the fan on the floor facing us now a deafening drone. Then Nonna said, in almost a whisper and almost lost to the din of the fans, "*Coraggio, Leeza. Coraggio.*"

Nonna was right. She should know about courage. Her life had been fraught with challenge, hardship and tragedy, all overcome or endured with courage—that same courage that was the foundation of her faith, positive attitude, love, resourcefulness and strong-willed determination. Her many stories and extraordinary examples contained valuable lessons unrecognized throughout my earlier years. The example-born lessons served as a lifesaving buoy to guide me, to keep me from drowning. The stories-born lessons were the rugged but solid Italian hill-climbing staff to lead me around obstacles and over hurdles.

It is Nonna's unshakable courage that lives within me and is the reason I survive to write this book.

Courage is:

- Believing you can succeed when others tell you cannot succeed.

- Believing you will be well when others say you will not be well.

- Having hope even if you think the situation may be hopeless.

Chapter 4

Old World Life Lessons in Courage for Nonna

A GREAT COMMOTION WAS OCCURRING IN THE RIZZO HOME. SAVERIA COULD hear the din all the way down the ancient, narrow, stone side street and into her grandmother's home. She was eight years old; old enough to know something significant was happening in the nearby home of her parents. She ran toward the loud shouting and cries, her long brown curls bouncing along behind her, highlighted red in the blazing Southern Italian sun.

"*Che l'è?*" (What is it Mama?) Saveria begged for an explanation, looking up as she pulled at her mother's gathered skirt.

Lezione Uno: Coraggio, Leeza (Lesson One: Courage, Lisa)

"*Una lettera da Zia Giulia in America!*" (A letter from Aunt Julia in America!) Her mother waived the letter in her hand as she exuberantly explained.

Her father picked up Saveria and twirled her around. *A celebration! Aunt Julia must send good news!* Word had come from Aunt Giulia in America. She had sent money for Saveria, her mother Giuseppina, her father Genaro and Saveria's two younger sisters to come to America.

Zia Giulia and her husband had left Calabria for America a couple years earlier. Saveria could no longer remember exactly how Zia Giulia looked, but heard Mother and Father talk about her often as they wondered when or *if* they might hear from her.

There was no means for Giuseppina and Genaro Rizzo to garner enough money to move their family to America. Genaro had spent the past several years as a World War I Italian soldier. His first daughter, Saveria, had not recognized her father when he returned for a brief furlough. Nine months after furlough, his second daughter was born. Genaro named her "Vittoria" (Victoria), to signify the victory he sought for Italy in the war. He would go on to valiantly risk his life in the November 1918 decisive battle of *Vittorio Veneto* (Victory at Veneto, Italy), successfully carrying ammunition by hand through the *Alte Vie* (high paths) long distance footpaths through the Dolomite Mountains of the Eastern Alps range. Genaro courageously darted through enemy fire to deliver the load to a group of artillery men who had been cut off from their allies and ammo. His bravery earned him a distinguished Medal of Honor, which he did not receive until 1984, almost a decade after he had died.

Back from the Alps to his beloved Giuseppina, a third child was conceived. As his band of Italian *soldati compare* (soldier buddies) pushed into Trieste it signified an important contribution to the end of World War I. Word reached Genaro in Trieste of the birth of a third daughter. In homage to the victory at Trieste and the fact that he survived the battles that led him to

Trieste, Genaro requested his third daughter be named *Triestina*.
Giuseppina agreed. Her *Zii*, (Italian aunts) believed the name ri-
diculously difficult and referred to her only as *Angelina* (angel), a
name that lingered for the rest of her life.

With the end of World War I, Genaro no longer had a soldier's salary but had four stomachs and his own to feed. Back in
Calabria, in the small town of Pedivigliano, Genaro was merely
a *mezzadro* (sharecropper). Genaro and Giuseppina rented one or
more *fico* (fig) trees. Giuseppina picked the deep purple succulent fruit, wrapped them in cloth, placed them in a willow basket
on top of her head and walked to markets in other villages. She
would walk up steep hillsides, through rivers, sometimes walking all night to reach a selling spot before a market would open
early the next morning. Genaro gathered slender limbs from the
willow trees during the summer. Through the winter he would
sit by the fireplace and weave a variety of willow baskets. The
baskets were also carried to market and sold. The money from
figs and baskets was barely enough to feed their family of five.
Perhaps a life in America would be better for us and our children,
Giuseppina had written to Zia Giulia to inquire about money for
voyage to America. Finally in April 1921, the letter from Aunt
Julia had arrived.

"*O Dio! Ringrazie a Dio!* (Oh God! Thanks to God!) Aunt Julia
had not forgotten us after all!"

Aunt Julia had sent enough money for an ocean passage for
all five and had filled out paperwork with the American government officials vouching to sponsor the family for a year.

Saveria jumped up and danced under the celebratory influence of the others in the small, dark, one room home. She did
not know her life was about to drastically change.

The events about to occur would set the stage for her to become my grandmother ... my *Nonna*.

The April evenings managed to cool, but the ever present,
rarely cloud-covered Southern Italian sun heated the day. Cars

and buses were unheard of and unimaginable to the residents of her small town of Pedivigliano, Calabria. Saveria's father arranged to rent a *triaino*, a small, rustic wood wagon pulled by a horse or mule to carry his three little girls and wife to Naples. He loaded the trunk that held their possessions: dresses for the girls and cloth-covered bundles of dried figs, bread and cheese. His wife was already seated in the front of the wagon and he handed her their baby daughter, Angelina. Just before he started out, he lifted his two older daughters onto the back of the wagon, Saveria, just eight years old and the oldest and her sister Vittoria, three years old. The little girls' legs dangled over the edge of the wagon bed as they sat with their backs to the horse and driver.

Little Vittoria was delighted at this new adventure ride. She started singing, "La, la, la, la, la, la lahhhh". Nonna would mimic the singsong decades later as she recalled the episode: the melody, a staccato version of the *Tarantella*, etched in her memory from the trauma of the event. Contrary to her sister's joyful singsong, Saveria was crying.

As was the custom in Southern Italy, the oldest granddaughter always was sent to live with the grandmother. True to custom, Saveria lived next door with her grandmother, precipitated by her father's return from World War I duty. Pedivigliano was nestled between hills, with tenacious crops grown ambitiously on the steep slopes. Most villagers had some type of makeshift garden on a plot of steep hillside. But water was very scarce and each family had one hour of water use per day with shifts assigned around the clock. Saveria's grandmother, Luisa Urso Masullo, had an assigned water use shift in the dead of night. In the bed they shared, her grandmother would gently tap her to wake for help with watering. Obediently, Saveria would rise and silently follow her grandmother thru darkened, steep, branch-covered paths on the walk to their garden. After they had arranged the log dams that shifted the water flow down the criss-crossing narrow irrigation channel to their plot of land, they would sit on the ground, listening to ensure the soft gurgle of rushing water. Her grandmother always carried a small meal for them. She would unwrap from linen cloths a chunk of *pane* (bread) and warm *castagni* (chestnuts) she had fished from her *fogoler* (open hearth) before departure. On the way home her grandmother would instruct Saveria to pick up any sticks or twigs her acute young eyes could spot from the light of the moon to burn in their hearth and provide warmth against the cool eve.

As the Rizzo wagon pulled away, Saveria sat facing her grandmother who stood in front of her grey, flat stone, mortar *casa*. Her grandmother was waving and crying out terms of endearment, stifled by insuppressible sobs. Saveria herself cried at leaving the grandmother she loved so dearly.

The wood wagon creaked and lurched from side to side as it passed over the stone and dirt road of Pedivigliano. Her sister Vittoria, in her adventure glee oblivious to the heart-wrenching separation scene around her, continued her *Tarantella* ditty. The creak of the wagon, Vittoria's singsong, and Saviera's cry was the melody of her departure from Pedivigliano.

Saveria's heart was broken as her grandmother disappeared in the distance. Her heart would break all over again when she told the story eighty years later. Her voice would crack from the tightness in her throat as she exclaimed that she never saw her beloved grandmother after that day. At the young age of eight, Saveria was embarking on a journey that would teach her the significance of courage.

The wagon slowly pulled them on the long journey through valleys and mountain passes of central Italy until they reached the seaside city of *Napoli* (Naples). This family lived their life, similar to most Italian families they knew, centered on an innate and deeply reverent faith. Genaro slowed the cart each time they passed the many *nicchia di ciglio della strada* (roadside grottos). Some appeared as five feet tall, open-faced, rectangular wood boxes, with statues of Jesus, Virgin Mary or a saint sheltered within. Some were more solidly constructed stone and mortar, arched grotto, enshrining a statue of a revered religious. There were long stretches of road where no structure or human was visible, yet seemingly from nowhere appeared the roadside grotto.

As a lighthouse beckons the ship safely to its destination, so did the *santuari* (sanctuaries) guide the Italian traveler on his spiritual and physical journey. The *santuari* were the connecting dots through which one could be guided, symbolic of the profound faith woven through the lives of Genaro, Giuseppina and their *compare* (close friends). Their eyes would fix upon a distant saintly dwelling. The cart would slow down as it passed, their eyes strained until the enshrined statue's benefactor was identified, and a silent prayer was uttered by each rider. Genaro would pray silently to the divine being for whom the shrine was dedicated: *Gesu, Sancta Maria, San Giuseppe* (Jesus, Holy Mary, Saint Joseph) *please guide me to Naples. Help me to know whether crossing to America is the correct decision for me and my family.* At the conclusion of his prayer, Genaro would place both the reins into the palm of one hand and respectfully make the Sign of the Cross with his free hand.

Giuseppina quietly murmured her prayer: *Gesu bambino, Madon, San Pietro* (Baby Jesus, Madonna, Saint Peter) *please protect my girls and my husband as we make our voyage to the United States.* Giuseppina shifted the weight of Baby Triestina in her arms to loosen one hand and reverently made the Sign of the Cross. Young Saveria, riding backward, would hear her mother's muffled prayer and turn her head in time to gape at the shrine. In imitation of her mother she made the Sign of the Cross and the cart jerked forward. *Gesu bambino, Madonna, I want to see my grandma.* Sister Vittoria, riding backward next to her, would in turn make the Sign of the Cross in the best-replicated reverence she was able as her little body jostled about. And thus traversed the *famiglia* (family) Rizzo toward an unknown and risky future, bolstered solely by a courage born of faith.

Zia Michelina, the sister of Giuseppina, lived in the sprawling city of Naples. Nothing had prepared Saveria for the sights she witnessed as her father tried to force the cart through the never-ending, narrow, crowded streets. Santuari were present, but the shrines were mere picture frames built flush into the façade of the building set back only three feet from the street. People pushed and shoved around vendors who called out the Italian names of live shellfish and recently alive fish they begged to sell.

The Rizzo family slept in the home of Zia Michelina the night before boarding their ocean liner, already parked in the *la baia di Napoli* (Bay of Naples). Giuseppina had a lot of news and future plans to discuss with her sister Michelina. With adults preoccupied, Saveria and her sisters crowded in the small closet. Saveria pulled the wood handle that dangled from a thin chain high above the bowl. She scrunched in fear as a loud swoosh of water came rushing from above into the toilet bowl. The three girls froze with astonishment and then released little girl giggles. Saveria repeated the magic again and again for her two sisters, standing next to the bowl wide-eyed with amazement. They had never before seen a toilet!

On April 10, 1921, Saveria trudged the steep incline of the wood boarding plank onto the Regina D'Italia ocean liner. The ship was bigger than any building she had ever seen! Near the top of the boarding plank she caught a glimpse through the handrail. Below her swarmed thousands of people. She studied individuals frantically trying to push their way through large huddled groups of anxious family members. Beyond the crowded dock were hundreds of boats; many sizes, many shapes, some moored to one of the dozens of docks, others gliding into or away from the magnificent Port of Naples.

Once on board, Nonna and her family were steered with crowds of about 1,900 other third class passengers to the lower decks. Unlike the first class passengers, there were up to two times the number of "steerage" passengers crammed into the same size cabin space. The space was no larger than a cargo hold. In fact, the space was used as cargo holds on the return trip from New York to Naples. Because they were considered "steerage" class, the men were separated from the women. Their tiny rooms had bunks stacked three and four high. When the ship hit an Atlantic storm, Saveria's mother Giuseppina and others on the ship became seasick.

More than seventy years later, when she was in her late eighties, Nonna appeared as a guest speaker in the classrooms of her great-grandsons and told the youngsters, entranced with fascination, about the transatlantic ocean liner trip. In her own words, she described the events:

> *The ship ran into a storm. It was supposed to take nine days to get to New York, but we ran into the storm and we had to stay below deck for three days. It was very sickening. Every one was getting sick. You would try to eat your food and try get up on deck, but you would throw up and down you would go again. The steps were full of beans and pasta. You didn't dare hang your head out of that bunk bed because you didn't know who was above you or when they would start to throw up.*

The storm and consequent seasickness were unrelenting. Saveria's mother was consumed by illness, but overwhelmed with concern for her three little girls, all of whom avoided seasickness. With all the focus she could muster her mother ordered the three girls to stay together in one bunk. Saveria would have to take charge.

"*Attenzione dall'alto!*" (Watch out from above!) Giuseppina sternly warned Saveria to keep her head and the heads of her sisters tucked within the bunk and be mindful of down-spouted vomit from the seasick occupants of above bunks.

The adult occupants of the tiny cabin room were all sick with no one to catch or carry pans of vomit. The occupants were so overcome by seasickness they could barely manage to lean their face over the bunk to vomit into the narrow space between the bunks. Saveria moved her two younger sisters against the wall and kept her own young body as the fortress against the showering vomit or falling onto the vomit-laden floor.

With great effort Giuseppina attempted to reach the ocean liner's deck to counter her seasickness and get her young girls out of the tiny sick room. "*Aria fresca, Saveria. Aria fresca, Saveria,*" (Fresh air, Sarah.) her mother repeated in determination.

By that time the climb above was a treacherous route because, not only were all of the floors swaying in response to the turbulent waters, they were also slippery with vomit. On deck, her mother leaned herself against the outside wall of a first class cabin room, took deep breaths of sea air, tried to hold her stomach and focused her vision on the horizon. She was so ill she could do nothing more than mutter a few instructions to Saveria. She relied on eight-year-old Saveria to be responsible for her two sisters.

Saveria felt the cool wet ocean air rushing against her cheeks as the ship cruised along at 14 knots. She saw endless dark blue waters over the top of the deck rail. Saveria was relieved to be out of the cramped smelly cabin into daylight and in *aria fresca*. She looked up at the two enormous yellow smoke stacks billowing smoke as black as the stripe around the top of the yellow funnel. She became entranced as she watched the people around her. Many were dressed differently than she had seen—women in fancy dresses with high tiny-buttoned boots and parasols; sailors in funny looking, tight, striped shirts and pants. She stared at two men who were conversing, but the words they were using she had never heard before. She tried to listen.

"*Saveria! L'bambina! Angelina!*" (Sarah! The baby! Angelina!)

Her mother's alarming cry jolted her. She looked at her mother who was pointing at a tiny ball wobbling away. Saveria's sister Angelina, not even having reached her first birthday, had chosen this moment to start to walk. But she didn't break into toddler milestone with baby steps; she started to run!

Some of the ocean liner crew were on deck for meal duty. The strong sailors carried wood crates stuffed with vegetables onto the deck. They stood some of the crates on an end and sat on them, using them as stools close to the deck rail and out of the walkway. Angelina spotted the crew sailors who sat against the deck rail cleaning bunches of lettuce for lunch and supper. *Fascinating! Enticing!* Off the proudly smiling tot went on a toddler's delighted dash toward the men. Mother Giuseppina yelled, "*Va via! Subito!*" (She is going away! Hurry!) for Saveria to hurriedly grab her little sister before she would run too close to the deck rail and hurtle into the ocean.

Saveria yelled to her baby sister, "*No! Fermate!*" (No! Stop!)

The effect of an older sister's command on a one-year-old's playful dash was a scream of glee and quest for freedom, and faster would her plump and bow-legged little legs go. For the first couple of runaway dashes, Saveria would calmly and responsibly recover and seat Angelina by her mother and sister Vittoria. Vittoria sat obediently at the folds of her mother's heavy wool skirt.

Saveria would pull down Angelina by the arm, seating her next to Vittoria, chiding, "*Unta montecare, a siede te qui*" (You sit here!).

But as soon as Saveria's back was turned, off Angelina would go toward the sailors!

"*Va via! Subito!*" (There she goes! Go immediately!)

Her mother would sound the alarm and off Saveria would go, chasing the escapee. It was a game now to her baby sister: chase her, grab her by the arm and drag her back. Well, the game grew tiring to Saveria. Upon the next return "I gave her a damn good bite on the arm!" as Nonna would tell it decades later. With a good bite for emphasis, "*A siede te. Unta montecare!*" she ordered. Angelina started to cry, but at least that kept her seated for a while. Saveria was in charge!

I think of the eight-year-old children I know these days, self-absorbed in expensive video games they have been given on demand, or pouting because they had to eat at the fast food restaurant their sibling requested and not the fast food place they wanted. I think of Nonna and how much courage and bravery it must have taken on her part to be separated from her dear grandmother, keep herself and her two infant sisters inside their small bunks and out of flying seasickness, and safe on the slippery deck of a ship overrun by strangers speaking unfamiliar languages.

As Nonna described close to a century later, "It didn't take long for the lice to take over the ship. The sinks and counters in the bathroom were so infested it looked as if they were moving and you had to blink and squint to see the movement was thousands of tiny lice."

Giuseppina tried desperately to protect her girls from lice infestation. The lice were multiplying exponentially each day. It was no use trying to wash out her girl's dresses in the lice-infested sinks. Instead, each day she would take out a new dress from their trunk and place it on her daughters. The dresses she had removed were already so laden with lice she would throw them overboard into the ocean.

Sixteen days after departure commotion ran through the ship. "*La stat di liberta! La stat di liberta!*", came the elated shouts as the Statue of Liberty was spotted. The masses ascended from the steerage holds and crowded the deck to view the renowned statue and symbol of the new world they were about to enter.

As the ship docked at Ellis Island, Giuseppina urged her husband, "Come on." "We have to be the first off this boat."

"Hold on", replied the honest Genaro. "I have to return the pots and pans. You remember? We were instructed when we boarded."

Indeed, when they boarded, Genaro was issued a set of tin pots, pans and eating utensils. As the male head of the family he was responsible to stand in line and obtain the meals. For steerage class, the meals, mostly *pasta fagiole* (pasta and beans), were doled into the pot of the person standing in line. The pot was carried to the long table where family waited and dished into individual pans from which each family member would eat. He brought lunch to his family and then washed the pots and pans so they would be clean for the dinner distribution.

"To hell with the pots and pans!"

True to the kind and gentle nature I remember of my Great-Grandfather Genaro, he obediently wanted to return the pots and dining utensils as instructed when issued to the family upon boarding.

"This ship is loaded with lice! We have to be the first off before the problem is discovered!" Giuseppina was emphatic and she rushed to put the remaining clean clothes on the family. The rest of their clothes she tossed overboard.

Giuseppina hurriedly bundled her family together and pushed them to the front of the line; Genaro was the seventh person in line, Saveria was the eighth. Giuseppina brought up the rear of the family, Vittoria in front of her and Angelina in her arms.

At the gangplank leading to American land they were visually inspected. The United States government inspector discovered no lice or other disease among the Rizzo family and the family was allowed to pass through to the Ellis Island arrival center. But when lice were discovered on a family behind them in line the United States immigration officials stopped the disembarking line.

The arrival center was crowded with people waiting for their loved ones to disembark the Italian ocean liner. Concerned, the waiting crowd began inquiring about the delay of Reg D'Italia ship passengers. Waiting themselves for immigration processing in the same room Genaro and Giuseppina overheard what had happened. The ship had been quarantined shortly after they had disembarked and eventually ended up being quarantined for forty days! But thanks to Giuseppina's quick thinking and determination, her family had been allowed off the ship.

Talk about courage. The Rizzo family had just survived a tumultuous transatlantic trip in a crowded ship plagued with vermin, with an infant and two little girls. But at that moment they needed to pull up another installation of courage. Not one of the five-member Rizzo family knew a word of English. They had passed the medical clearance portion of immigration processing by hand motion miming and complete acquiescence on the ship's gangplank. They stood on the vast worn floor of the Great Hall immigration area of Ellis Island. They glanced up toward the high painted ceiling and fought the urge to become overwhelmed among the mass of humanity with no means of communicating to another soul. But they had determination born of courage and courage born of faith. They had made it this far and believed they could accomplish the immigration processing and make their way to Zia Giulia.

Two U.S. immigration workers smiled as they hand-motioned to the Rizzo family and pinned tags on their shirts. From the workers' gestures they guessed the tags named their destination: Detroit. The aide women at Ellis Island guided the Rizzo family to the correct train that would take them to Detroit.

The excitement of the train diminished as the tiny tummies of the three little sisters began to growl with hunger. The Rizzo family had no food with them. They had not eaten since their last meal on the ship. The girls began crying to their mama, "*Sei mun comati, sei mun comati*" (We are hungry! We need something to eat!) Two people seated in front of the Rizzo family made gestures indicating a willingness to share food they had packed. Embarrassed because they did not even know how to say "yes" or "no", the parents ignored the generous couple. The famished girls quieted for a few minutes but returned to their pleading. Soon thereafter, the train steward, with assorted snacks on a tray, reached the Rizzo's row of seats. Genaro reached into his pocket and held out a palm displaying American coins. The train steward took some coins and gave each of the three teary-eyed girls a candy bar. Saveria had never seen a packaged candy bar. She tore away the crinkly paper and bit off a piece. The flavors were more rich and exotic than the fig or orange treats she experienced in her grandmother's home!

Not one more complaint was uttered by Saveria for the continuance of her high-speed traverse from New York City to Detroit.

As with many homeowners in their eastside Detroit neighborhood, Zia Giulia had a boarder who paid a modest amount to sleep in an upstairs room and partake of family meals. Even better than the rent income, the boarder owned a car. With a flurry of excited anticipation Zia Giulia slid into the passenger seat and with both arms gesturing "*Andiamo! Presto!*" she ordered the boarder-driver to the Grand Trunk railroad station.

The Grand Trunk railroad station was the most magnificent multi-story building in southwest Detroit. Hundreds of people crowded the cavernous lobby bustling to and from the train platforms. Zia Giulia immediately recognized her niece Giuseppina amid the crush of people exiting the train. With a loud cry the women rushed together for an animated embrace. After a kiss to both of Giuseppina's tear-stained cheeks and a pinch to the cheeks of each her tiny wide-eyed grandnieces, she ushered the Rizzo family into the boarder's car. A car!

Saveria had never before ridden in a car! With an American candy bar delighting her tummy, she was speeding along in a car faster than she had ever moved before. She looked down. The road whizzing by beneath her was not stone and dirt, but was smooth pavement! She looked up and saw many buildings taller than the tallest building she knew in *Pedivigliano,* the *SS Pietro e Paolo* church in the center of town. Some of the houses were made of wood, not the stacked flat rock of her parent's and grandmother's home.

At eight years of age, Saveria, my Nonna had endured the adventure to her new home in Detroit, Michigan in the United States of America and learned about courage along the way. She endured the tragic departure from her beloved grandmother, helped her young sisters survive a tumultuous ocean crossing, and embraced arrival in a strange land with undecipherable language and custom.

With mismatched Salvation Army clothes and shoes so ill-fitted they frequently flipped off her feet, little Saveria bravely and enthusiastically walked to the Detroit public grade school. She did not understand a word of what was spoken by her teachers or classmates, yet she sat eagerly and proudly each day. Courage!

My Nonna, would repeatedly return to her cache of courage when faced with struggles that appeared throughout her long life.

Now, seven decades after her unwanted exodus from Italy, I was lying alone in a nursing home almost a continent away from Nonna. I thought of how she had attempted to pass along the strength and determination garnered from a life of difficult lessons. "*Coraggio, Leeza. Coraggio,*" I could hear her whisper the words in my ear.

Could I truly muster the bravery needed to get me through my current nursing home situation?

So much had happened since the infamous rheumatoid arthritis diagnosis five years ago. So much had gone wrong. Terribly, terribly wrong.

Courage is:

- Taking charge of any possible aspect of an overwhelming situation.
- Taking action even when you are afraid.
- Searching every adverse situation to find the lesson held within.
- Making an attempt even though you believe it is too difficult to change.

CHAPTER 5

This Can't Be Happening to Me!

MY SUMMER CALCULUS COURSE CONCLUDED AND I RECEIVED THE HIGHEST number of grading points in the class by a significant margin. *See? You can make it in medical school. The family doctor is the fool, not you.* I had about six weeks until my Junior year classes began at Aquinas College in Grand Rapids, Michigan. My sister Laura had just graduated from the all-girl Catholic Dominican High School in Detroit. Laura and I started talking about moving to Los Angeles, California where our mother lived, and my mother kicked into high gear to entice and prepare for our arrival.

I continued to hold a deep and mostly unrecognized resentment against my mother for secretly walking away from our family on Christmas Eve 1975. But deep within, I was delighted to be reunited with her; not that I would ever show her my delight while she was alive, a naïve mistake that would haunt me the rest of life. Nonetheless, this high energy, persuasive woman performed astonishing back-flips to ensure Laura would be enrolled that Fall semester in the comparatively tuition-free California State University system. And with assured resolve she adeptly cleared hurdles to enroll me in the prestigious all women's Mount Saint Mary's College high in the mountains over Los Angeles.

My mother's enthusiasm and gratitude for the Mount Saint Mary enrollment was emphasized as she drove me for dorm move-in day and my first view of the campus. She turned her white Gremlin hatchback off Sunset Drive to head through the residential Brentwood streets to the mountain top campus, her arms outstretched to excitedly grasp the steering wheel, smile stretched just about as far as arms.

"Oh Lisey! You won't believe how gorgeous Mount Saint Mary's is! It is truly part of God's heaven on earth!"

The older little white Gremlin had to work against an almost vertical angle as we grew closer to the hilltop campus. It was barely chugging now.

From the sputtering, gasping and jerking, I was becoming doubtful whether the car and my few possessions would succeed in arriving at hilltop. "Is the car going to make it?"

"You betcha! We're almost there!" she responded to me, and then to the car, "C'mon my precious baby. You can do it. I know you can!"

She patted the blue plastic dashboard as if stroking a beloved old workhorse. The car jerked forward a few more yards. The thought crossed my mind, *Boy, it's as if it is her sheer optimism and enthusiasm that is fueling the car, willing it to the top!*

Lezione Uno: Coraggio, Leeza (Lesson One: Courage, Lisa)

We passed through the gates announcing our arrival at the home of the Sisters of Saint Joseph of Carondelet, the road ahead again vertical, lined with elegantly thin and tall eucalyptus trees.

"C'mon baby; just a little more!" But this time my mother did not pat precious baby's dash, the road too steep to remove her hands from the steering wheel.

We pulled into Chalon Circle, the heart of the campus. My breath was lost in a gasp as my heart soared. It was almost too exquisite, too close to paradise to believe. *We have reached Heaven!*

"And look, Mother Mary is greeting us."

Sure enough, at the opposite side of the Chalon Circle drive was a pure white statue of the Blessed Virgin Mary. The college Patroness' stark white composition imbued the purity and chasteness for which she is renowned, her arms outstretched as if to embrace me and whisper in my ear, *Welcome to this sacred setting. I will safeguard and love you all the days you make this your dwelling place.*

It was an incredibly moving moment to see Mother Mary in this pastoral setting and feel the heart-given salutation. Blessed Mary, the Christian symbol of humility and love through the sorrows her life bore, had taken a maternal, nurturing role after my mother had left Michigan five and a half years ago.

"C'mon, I want to show you some of the spectacular views!"

In unspoken tandem we both left the car and headed toward Mother Mary. We were drawn to her with a deep sense of gratitude-born obligation; to stand before her in awe and gratitude that I had actually made it across the continent to this magical setting where I would continue my education toward medical school.

Before any further act we would devote this moment in this unparalleled spiritual place to pay homage and thanksgiving to God. After a minute of head-bent, reverent silence

I felt my mother place her hands on my shoulders. She slowly turned my body 180 degrees. *Magnifico!* (Magnificent!) For the second time in a matter of minutes my breath was stopped by a panorama of remarkable beauty. The cloudless, pale-blue Southern California sky met the deep blue rippling waters of the Pacific Ocean. Catalina Island dotted the ocean's horizon. To the right were Mediterranean style homes tucked into the hillsides of Brentwood and Santa Monica. To the left downtown Los Angeles skyscrapers were visible through a thin layer of dingy brown smog. At our feet lay the Campus Circle drive bordered in part by a covered walkway with arched columns, perfectly edged green and flowered landscaping, and red-tiled buildings in which I would be residing and drinking in knowledge.

"See, Honey Bunny? Isn't this glorious? Isn't this just simply glorious? Oh, thank you God!"

I merely kept nodding my head in acquiescence. It was stunning to take in beauty as I had never seen before while simultaneously realizing the setting was going to be my home for the next several years. The multiple and overwhelming feelings had momentarily muted me. Apparently the location had overwhelmed many others; the Chalon Circle was the backdrop familiar to many Hollywood productions including Mel Brooks' "High Anxiety", "Less Than Zero" and the high school in "The O.C." television series."

Prior to Laura's and my arrival in California, my mother had moved her mother, my *Nagymama,* into a small modular home nestled among pungent wild rosemary bushes and arid mountains in the canyon below Malibu. My grandfather, *Nagypapa,* had died the year before from prostate cancer. So it was a fond reunion of three generations of women.

My mother and *Nagymama,* of Hungarian royalty, had regal posture and long elegant legs leading toward six feet in height. My blond-haired, blue-eyed, sparking-smile mother was stunningly beautiful. My sister, too, inherited the long gorgeous legs and beautiful Italian features, recognized quickly as she won the coveted Miss Cal State Northridge award within months of arriving on campus. A not so flattering set of Italian genes expressed themselves dominantly in me—shorter-legs and larger nose. It was not very bothersome to be the less-beauteous of the group. Besides, I was quietly initiating steps toward entering religious life as a nun. I was amused by all the extravagant tactics men would take to impress my mother and sister, at the same time relieved I did not have to undergo the same pressures.

My mom sang professionally, a soprano voice so pure and full I could sit transfixed listening to her for hours. It harkened me back to my childhood where it was normal course to sing in harmony or in rounds at home, in the car, at campfires, and at parties pretty much all the time. My mother was the lead of course. Nagymama was quick to join in an alto harmony. My specialty was the soprano descant; I couldn't wait to perch my high notes above the others. Laura would join in any of the three parts or one of her own. The quartet was reunited again after almost a decade.

My mother would give anything, even her own health, to restore my health and rid me of rheumatoid arthritis. The traditional medical regiments were barely touching the disease. She discovered every imaginable alternative healer, made appointments, picked me up from college, drove me and took notes during the appointments. Any purported curative diet that hit her radar she bought the products. Soon I was faithfully adhering. She often worked four to five jobs at a time to help pay for the healers and products. But nothing was working to slow the assault. The disease was cruelly and rapidly ravishing any joint it chose. My youthful rebellion had fueled my determination to finish undergrad despite the nay-saying of the diagnosing doctor.

As the end of my last semester approached I had no cartilage left in my knee joints. When I tried to stand from a seated position, from across the room was heard the cracking and popping of the knee as the bones ground against each other without benefit of smooth cartilage. On several occasions, people around me would stop and stare in disbelief or horror at the sound and recognition of the cause. The pain was tremendous when trying to walk, even short distances.

Most frightening to me was the loss of stamina. I pushed myself to finish senior exams. After my last exam, instead of blasting my stereo, packing and enjoying joyful exchanges with friends passing in the hall as everyone else, I collapsed on my narrow dormitory bed. I remember opening my eyes and seeing my mother and my friend Maria, putting my few belongings into boxes. I tried to lift my head but felt alarmingly weak, gave in to a feeling of fainting, and closed my eyes again. I opened them when sensing my mother above me, carefully taking down and wrapping the reproduction of the *Botticelli's* Virgin Mary she had given me as a gift. She had hung the *Botticelli* Mary above my bed nine months earlier to inspire my final year of undergrad. I turned my pillowed head from my mother and saw Maria sweeping my dorm room floor. I closed my eyes again to keep the room from spinning. *What is happening to me?*

In this declining physical state, I moved in with my mother and grandmother. My mother had secured a three-bedroom apartment in the upscale Warner Park area of Woodland Hills. I would have my own room, Mom and Nagymama would share another, and the third would be for a roommate who could help pay the rent.

Despite my mother's and grandmother's loving devotion, I did not regain strength. I explained to my mother that I felt as if I only had "one toe remaining on this earth." I expressed to her I was sorry, but did not know if I would be able to stay on earth much longer. I gathered every bit of energy and sent out medical school applications. I had to get into medical school. It was my life's passion. It would propel me to determined wellness.

Soon, the medical school secondary requests for information fell to the wayside. I was drawn into deep sleep for 18 to 20 hours a day. I awoke to use the commode placed next to my bed and called to my Nagymama or mother to come and empty it. During the most ill period, I could not sit up for the commode and they placed a bedpan beneath me. The least painful was to remain lying on my side, curled in the fetal position.

My mother would arise at 5:45 a.m. and retrieve from the refrigerator the carrots Nagymama had selected from the 20-pound bag of organic carrots and had scrubbed clean the night before. Mom would grind the carrots in the expensive state-of-the art juicer and bring the sweet, thick-orange, healing liquid to my room. She would pull up the window blinds and would sweetly whisper, "Good morning honey bunch!"

My elbows were frozen in the bent position, too painful to unlock and extend, let alone to hold a 12-ounce glass of liquid. My mother would lift my head with one hand and gently hold the glass of carrot juice to my lips with her other hand. When she returned much later in the day, she and Nagymama would take me by wheelchair into the bathroom, transfer me onto the shower bench and shower me. I think back and recognize how enormously these two women loved me: Nagymama scrubbing carrots every night; Mom having to drag herself from bed after only five hours of sleep; devotedly toileting and showering their adult daughter/granddaughter; the endless hours of beseeching prayers for my healing, all performed with the desperate hope that their actions and prayers would produce a cure from the vicious rheumatoid arthritis that besieged their beloved Lisa.

Courage is:

- Providing care for an ill or dying person even though you feel uncomfortable, frustrated, exhausted or hopeless.

- Graciously accepting care from another when you are too ill to care for yourself.

- Leaving the comfort zone for a healthier lifestyle.

- Continuing to fight for what you believe and hope, even when it appears the world is falling in around you.

- Stepping into your day even though your body hurts too much to move.

- Smiling throughout your day even though your body hurts too much to smile.

CHAPTER 6
The Accident

TWO YEARS PASSED LIVING UNDER THE FERVENT CARE OF MY MOTHER AND Nagymama and I was feeling stronger. I had not taken even one step in those two years, but I was strong enough to slowly use my dangling feet to maneuver the wheelchair around the apartment. If I angled and positioned myself carefully I could squeeze myself in the wheelchair into the narrow bathroom and configured a way to transfer onto the toilet seat or the shower chair. *Oh the joy of bathroom privacy*! Unless you have had the prolonged experience of having other people carry your every bodily excretion in a pan for disposal, you may not fully understand the intensity of appreciation for returning to bathing and toileting independently.

Christmas 1986 was to arrive in a couple of days and plans were made for a road trip to Montana for the Christmas holiday. My mother and Nagymama were contemplating a move there and would check out a new home during the trip. A few days before the trip we discussed the possibility of me not going. To be honest, I was not thrilled about the long car trip to cold environs, but my mother could not bear the thought of me being alone on Christmas Eve and Christmas Day. The more Montana Christmas cold weather gear that was packed into the car, the more evident my wheelchair would not fit. My mother found a mutual friend who planned to remain in Los Angeles and who would also be away from family on Christmas. The friend told us she would be glad to stay with me over the holiday and promised that we would have fun together.

Two days before Christmas Eve there was the flurry of last minute packing. My mother had been working several jobs at one time, sleeping only four to five hours a night in order to earn enough money to take days off for the vacation and to afford the travel expenses. Mom and Nagymama were behind schedule. They had wanted to depart for Montana hours earlier.

Suppertime was fast approaching. The kitchen pots were in a lower cupboard where I could reach. I fished around in the refrigerator for vegetables and threw them into a small pot of boiling ramen noodles so all three of us could have soup for a meal.

Mom commented the soup was "Mmmm, good!" as she walked around, slurping from her bowl and trying to remember to pack last minute items. "You take such good care of me, Lisa." The words spoken were with the tenderness of an affectionate mother. She, who devoted so much of her time to taking good care of me whereas I had only concocted a measly, watery soup.

As a last preparation before departure, my mother brought out my decoratively wrapped Christmas presents. She set them in front of the fake fireplace, the type we could plug in and watch the plastic grey log glow orange from a light bulb hidden within. She gave an animated description of the fun we would have opening Christmas presents together when she returned. She had decorated the mantel of the fake fireplace with pine boughs she had gathered from the ground where the Christmas tree merchant departed after selling all his trees. She wrapped a wide purple satin ribbon around the boughs and interspersed miniature gold Christmas bulbs. After marriage and while raising four children, Mom had obtained an Associate Degree in fine arts from the community college and artistry flowed from her. She was a master at taking a simple item or another person's cast away and creating beauty from it. Our living room, festive and smelling of Christmas thanks to her golden touch was now further adorned by presents.

Mom stood after arranging the presents around the fireplace and moved toward the door. I rolled my wheelchair close to her, pulled out a sealed Christmas card and gave it to her. I had spent a lot of time trying to find the right words to include in the card and I wanted her to have it now. I told her I wanted her to take it with her so she could open it on Christmas Eve, read it, and feel my presence. She was standing in the walkway outside our apartment now. A smile shone on her face at the gesture.

She turned toward me, her smile dimming and said softly, "Pray for me, Lisa." She looked deep into my eyes, pleading seriously, "Pray for me *really* hard."

I was not exactly sure why or for what she wanted me to pray. I saw her tuck the card into her large, bulging purse as she bent to kiss me good-bye on the cheek. *Dear God, she looks tired.*

Less than two hours after their departure, I heard the muffled but desperate voice of the "promise to spend the holidays with me and have fun" friend. *It sounded as if she was on the phone with an airline company. Was she trying to find a last minute flight home to her family for Christmas? It could not be. She just promised Mom she would stay here with me.* The few minutes warning helped to prepare me. Thus, it was not a shocking surprise when she approached me apologetically, stumbling to find the right words saying she knew she had promised my mother and me that she would accompany me for Christmas.

"I realized I could not be away from family for Christmas. I actually found a flight that leaves in a few hours. It has several stop-overs, but I will be at my parent's home by Christmas Eve."

The promised Christmas friend left shortly thereafter, and with her departure was every plan I had for a Christmas Eve and Christmas Day celebration with another human being. Mom and Nagymama and my friends all thought I was nicely situated and spoken for. In this pre-cell phone era there was no means of reaching Mom and Nagymama during their two-day long drive. *No need to be mopey. No need to interfere with any of your friends' family plans. You don't want Mom or Nagymama to worry or turn around. It is only two celebrated days. It's okay if you don't celebrate on the actual Christmas Eve and Christmas Day. The celebration will be postponed until Mom gets back next week. Then you can celebrate Christmas, just the two of you for the first time in your life. That will be special! You can stick it out alone for now.*

With the departure of the promised Christmas friend was also the ability to reach any object above or outside my seated position in the wheelchair along with the capability to leave the apartment. *Uh-oh. You can't even maneuver the wheelchair over the doorstop to get out of the apartment. What happens if you fall onto the ground? You won't be able to get up or get to a phone to call for help and no one will be checking in until Mom gets back in a week. Stop it, Lisa. You are tough. You are clever. You'll figure out how to make it work.*

The next morning was the day before Christmas Eve. It was the first day since I had moved in that I had ever been alone in the three-bedroom apartment. But I did not mind. Instead I took advantage of the solitude by taking an extra long, hot shower. I usually had Mom or Nagymama help me from my wheelchair onto the shower chair in the tub. But I was determined to be clean for my solo Christmas Eve, and with my physics lessons bolstering strategy and several grunts of physical effort I made it onto the shower bench, shuddered and yelped through the first few minutes of frigid water, then smiled, face-forward into the stream as the warm water engulfed me and alleviated my aching joints.

What a glorious way to prepare for Christmas Eve! Steam and massaging water; surrounding, cleansing, soothing. No rush to make way for the next person to shower. It was the perfect backdrop for an operatic performance. I could feel it coming, building from my heart into my larynx and within a fragment of time I was blissfully lost in my own renditions of *Ah! Sweet Mystery of Life at Last I Found Thee.*

My mother and I had watched the 1935 MGM musical *Naughty Marietta* just a week before and the chorus of its signature song continued to rattle around my brain. Jeanette McDonald and Nelson Eddy at their best!

> *Ah! Sweet Mystery of Life, at last I've found thee,*
> *Ah! I know at last the secret of it all.*
> *All the longing, seeking, striving, waiting, yearning,*
> *The idle hopes, the joy and burning tears that fall!*
>
> *For 'tis love and love alone, the world is seeking,*
> *And 'tis love and love alone, I've waited for!*
> *And my heart has heard the answer to its calling,*
> *For it is love that rules forever more!*

It was quite the diva shower concert!

Ah----Sweet My-ster-y of life …

… as loudly as I wanted, the enclosed shower a perfect echo chamber, knowing I would not disturb anyone.

And--- tis love- and love - a-lone, I've waited for …

… in the highest range possible to stretch my vocal cords, knowing I could not shame myself by being overheard.

I tried singing it to emulate Jeannette McDonald's melodious voice, forcing sound through pinched nostrils and picturing myself cooing to the powder-faced Nelson Eddy. I chuckled when I thought about how my mother and I had looked at each other during the closing duet scene. Mercenary Eddy, the dashing, dynamic Captain Richard Warrington, had bravely rescued McDonald, the feisty French Princess Marietta, from pirates. After an hour and a half of feigned dislike for one another they serenaded each other at realized ardor. The beautiful but stubborn princess swooned by a rescuer, forceful but enamoring. *Sigh.* I sniffled. I turned to look at my mother, staring engrossed at the small TV screen, eyes filled with tears. *Boy, we are suckers for sap.* She must have had the exact thought. Simultaneously we looked at each other's sentimental state and burst out giggling. How silly we were at becoming emotional over an over-dramatic scene where the delicate Jeanette McDonald gazed longingly into a powder-faced, high and thinly-plucked eyebrow Eddy, an image not exactly conjuring romance.

My thoughts drifted from recalling movie night to the present. *I wonder how the traveling is going for Mom and Nagymama. How far had she driven before she had to pull over to rest for the night? Were they getting close to their destination?* It was 1986, years before anyone in my family would have a cell phone. My mother told me she would call me when they arrived at their destination in Montana. I did not expect to hear from her until then.

Lord, keep them safe. Angels, surround their car. Guide them. Protect them.

I transferred from my wheelchair to my twin bed, hoping to trap some of the warmth from the shower by snuggling under the covers. I was exhausted. It had been an energy expending endeavor to undress, get in and out of the shower, towel dry, and redress, all without being able to stand, limited by painfully contracted arms. I laid my head back on the pillow.

The phone next to my bed rang.

Lezione Uno: Coraggio, Leeza (Lesson One: Courage, Lisa)

"I'm calling about Anna Barczay." said a woman with an older sounding voice and a slight regional drawl I could not place. "Do you know her?" The woman sounded serious.

"Yes. Anna Barczay is my grandmother. What about her?" I asked.

"I am a volunteer with the Fillmore Community Hospital in Utah." was the response. "I need to give you some information. Is there someone there with you, dear?" asked the woman in a compassionate tone.

"No." I replied. I was alarmed. Nagymama was approaching her 70s, but she was as strong and healthy as an ox. *Had Nagymama become ill during the trip? I'm sure Mom is with her somewhere in the hospital. Knowing Mom she doesn't want to leave Nagymama's side and asked this obliging volunteer to call me. Whatever it is do not let this woman hang up without telling me what is going on with Nagymama!*

I was sitting upright in my bed now on full alert.

"I am the only one here. I am pre-med, worked as a medical volunteer and have applied to medical school so I am accustomed to dealing with medical issues. It is okay to tell me right now."

I spoke authoritatively, stopping myself short of pleading.

You have to convince her to tell you what is happening. You can't let her hang up. Who knows how long it will be before Mom can break away and call. And what if Mom needs you to do something to help, even if to pray.

The woman hesitated.

C'mon lady! Just tell me! Even though in reality it was probably a few seconds, I could not bear it. I feared what she might tell me but I feared more her hanging up. I had never heard of Fillmore. There was no such thing as Internet research and I was alone without a way out of an apartment.

"Well," she started with trepidation. "There has been a serious car accident. Anna is in the emergency room right now. The doctors know she has a broken pelvis that will need surgery but they are not sure of the extent of her internal injuries."

Oh no! Poor sweet Nagymama! Lord be with her. Help her!

"So, will they be able to do the surgery soon? Can they look for the internal injuries during the surgery?" The innate doctor in me had kicked in.

"Anna's pelvis is actually shattered. The doctor's are concerned one of the sharp bone fragments might puncture the major arteries located in the area. That can be serious. So they will look first at the shattered pelvis fragments and secure any arteries. They want to do this right away, so they are prepping her now for immediate surgery. They can tell more about other possible internal injuries once they get her into surgery."

It sounded serious, but there was also hope.

Lord, Let every surrounding artery be unharmed.

"Okay. Yes. Please get her into surgery as soon as possible."

As I gave her permission for the doctors to perform emergency surgery, it dawned on me, *why is she asking me for permission? Mom is there. She can give consent to surgery.* Maybe the woman wasn't calling to get permission from me; maybe just to let me know while Mom was at Nagymama's gurney, holding her hand and speaking gentle reassuring words in her native Hungarian language.

Wait a minute. Why hasn't she mentioned anything about Mom? The car accident. What about the car accident? What about Mom?

Fighting to keep my voice from cracking, I asked, "Where is Julia Barczay? Julia is my mother. Is it possible to speak to my mother?"

"Is there any friend or family close by that you can call to come be with you?" was the calm response. But it was a non-response.

My thoughts raced even faster. I could feel my heart pounding so hard it was thumping against my chest.

"Yes. I have a friend that can be here in a minute."

"Why don't you call your friend? I will call you back in a few minutes."

But I need to know <u>now</u>.

"Where is Julia?"

I was firm, demanding. Silence followed the demand. Had she hung up on me for being too pushy? Maybe it was the blood pulsing through my head from pounding heart, muffling my hearing?

"Julia is dead." came the short response.

What? Julia dead? IMPOSSIBLE!

Julia was the one full of life; perpetually exuding light and high energy. My racing thoughts began crashing into one another. Mom's driver license must have become confused with Nagymama's identification card. Yeah. That's what it was. In the jostle and tumult of the accident, however it had occurred, their purses had spilled open and IDs had become switched.

"I'm sorry. You must be mistaken. Julia is the young one. Her mother is Anna the older one."

Immediately after the words had spilled from my mouth I realized what I had said. Guilt stabbed at me.

Oh, dear Jesus. Please forgive me. What have I just said? I didn't mean that I wanted Nagymama to be dead. She was my dear, stately, loving grandmother. Please don't let her be dead. It is just that Julia ... Mom ... can't be dead. Oh God. She just can't be dead!

Both women were physically and emotionally strong. They were fighters and survivors. They had survived fleeing from their homeland and living in refugee camps of World War II, for heaven's sake. Nagymama, in her seventies, had a slim, toned body with a keen intelligent mind. My mother had a college degree in physical education. She was only 48 and her athletic ability could put people half her age to shame. It was not feasible, utterly impossible that these vibrant, tough, World War II survivors could have the life snuffed out on a mere holiday trip!

"Yes. Julia is the younger one. She was pronounced dead at the scene of the accident. I ... I understand it was a terrible accident. The car rolled several times." (Pause.) "It happened in a rural area outside of Kanosh. They brought Anna here to our hospital in Fillmore because it was the closest hospital. I'm very sorry, dear."

Racing, crashing thoughts slam-halted as I hung up the phone. I only had a single thought now. *I can't live … if living is without you, Mom! You are my best friend... everything to me. I need you, Mom! I cannot live without you!* The words moving across my mind were a ticker tape in a recurring cycle.

I was repeating the thought aloud now, over and over. "Mom! Mom! Where are you Mom? I cannot live without you! Can't you hear me? I cannot live without you! *You are my everything. I need you, Mom!* "

I was choking out the protestations in sobs. I started shouting the call, even though no one was in the apartment, even though my mother did not answer from this world or the next.

The cries subdued to repeated moans: "Oh God. Oh God. Oh God … "

I switched from talking aloud to my Mom to talking aloud with God. It was "Negotiating with God" time. "God, for years I have prayed every day that if you just allow me to swing my legs out of bed each morning, stand and walk, I would devote my whole life to serving you. I will give up that desire to walk now. I will stay in the wheelchair the rest of my life, but please, please, PLEASE GOD … do not let Mom be dead. I will even give up medical school. My dream of medical school I will give up just to have Mom alive. Please, God. PLEASE!"

She had asked me to pray for her. *As she walked away from you for the last time, she turned back, looked you in the eyes and added:* "Pray. Pray REALLY hard!"

But … instead of praying you had been singing some frivolous MGM song in the shower. Oh, Lisa.

Did the song have any significance to what had just occurred? Ah! *Sweet Mystery of Life, at last I've found thee … it is love that rules forever more!*

Lezione Uno: Coraggio, Leeza (Lesson One: Courage, Lisa)

My mother and I both believed in miracles; in metaphysical occurrences standard science could not explain. We were closely and uniquely emotionally and spiritually connected to one another. If she had really just died, how come I had not sensed her danger or her passing? What about all those stories of emotionally and soul-tied relationships where at one person's peril or death, the other's aligned soul twinged with the sensation of what occurred. It would have happened to us, too because I knew we were that close. It added ache to my hurting soul to acknowledge I had no otherworldly sense of my mother's passing. No beyond-this-realm communication to me that she was okay or that she parted with undying love for me. I had nothing but a cruel, aching, cold void.

It hurt badly inside. It hurt so that I could not sleep. Someone called my doctor and got me a sleeping pill, but the pill didn't work. My dreams were possessed by a frantic search for my mother, and still, from those midnight terrors, I had to wake up. To wake meant consciousness. In the waking moments before consciousness kicked in I felt a dull, crushing ache in my gut. And then conscious thought brought reality and I remembered what had happened.

Then my daytime nightmare would begin. My face was on that same pillow my mother would bend over when returning late at night from her second or third job of the day. She would softly kiss me on the cheek and tuck the covers under my chin. I could feel the warmth of her cheek and smell her perfume even now. Sure I was an adult in my early twenties and sure this was my mother giving me a good night kiss. At the time I sometimes snubbed her attempt at goodnight sentiment, residual resentment from her leaving the family years ago, and would turn my face away. It felt like a kick in the gut to think I could have been so cruel, to realize I squandered a precious gift of love. Now I longed to feel that tender endearment just one last time.

Why hadn't I gone on the trip and been in that car too? If I would have been in the car I, too, would be dead and wouldn't have to feel the crushing pain of devastating loss right now.

Julia was all light, all joy; a gift to so many. I was merely a crippled girl, a burden to others.

Courage is:

- Loving again after you have been hurt by others.
- Loving again after the loss of a beloved.

CHAPTER 7

Neurotransmitter Imposters

THE DAYS FOLLOWING THE FATEFUL PHONE CALL WERE BLURRED IN A SWIRL of shock, heartache and grief. Emotional and physical stresses were treacherously mounting. I was on the phone constantly engaged in emotional conversations as I related the horror over and over to the multitude of my mother's and grandmother's friends and family, frustrated by attempts to make post-death arrangements from the confinement of a wheelchair for a body undergoing autopsy out-of-state, or keeping tabs on Nagymama in a Utah intensive care unit.

My mother's magnetic personality fostered friendships all around the world. How could I possibly notify every friend and family member? How could a funeral service be arranged to accommodate the number and diversity of friends and family? The Utah County coroner could not even promise when her body or ashes might be released for delivery to California. My sister and two brothers were in Michigan, it was Christmas, the busiest airline travel time of the year and there were scarce few flights available.

From my wheelchair in the apartment I made arrangements for a memorial service to be held at my mother's church for her church community the day after Christmas. Although it would be held only three days after her death, I was glad the hectic rush would consumedly plow me through Christmas. I planned a second service which would be held in the Chapel at Mount St. Mary's College for family and friends who were not church members, and for my friends. My mother loved Mount St. Mary's College campus and she was overjoyed that I could attend school there. I then worked on arrangements for my brothers and sister to fly from Michigan to Los Angeles in time for both services.

In addition to the non-stop death notification and post-death arrangements, it seemed an insurmountable task to write and deliver a tribute for the memorial services. What could I say to ever capture a person who was so vivaciously alive? How do you describe a person who had a significant positive effect on many lives?

Jozsef Cardinal Mindszenty, an icon for my mother and many Hungarian Freedom Fighters, delivered a sermon in Hungary forty-one years prior to the date of the my mother's death. Three years after proclaiming his sermon on December 23, 1945, the Hungarian Cardinal was arrested by the Soviets and forced into solitary confinement for eight years. In his sermon, Cardinal Mindszenty used Apostle John's phrase, "God is love" (I John 4:8):

> *Anyone who is full of hate does not belong to Christ, nor can he be a complete human being. Only through love can a human being reveal his true worth; only through love can he overcome himself.*

Lezione Uno: Coraggio, Leeza (Lesson One: Courage, Lisa)

The teachings of St. John and my mother's mentor, Cardinal Mindszenty, seemed to flow perfectly and miraculously into the tribute for my mother. When it came time for the eulogy someone pushed my wheelchair and positioned me facing the participants next to a 24-inch-by 36-inch photo of my mother in her teen years:

> *Julia had reached her goal of self-desirelessness and so emptied herself of human imperfection that she could only be filled with God. She could be totally filled with that God love that she so yearned for. That was ever present upon her lips and in her prayers and divine calls. That is what Julia wants for all of us, too, to fill ourselves with God's love and her love which is now part of His. She would pray at least an hour each morning before she started her day and again in the evening before going to sleep. She also put some of her heavenly requests into writing. On Christmas morning, one of her last written prayer requests was found. It started by saying, "The desire of my heart is to serve you twenty-four hours a day. That my family be taken care of. To serve by ministering unto people, helping them, singing to them." On the backside of that note were the only and final words: "Serve in Joy until ..." We now know that her prayers were answered. The words that so many people use to describe her are: Joy, Love, Giver and Beauty. She indeed was the dawn of each day; a beam of light and joy in all of our lives. Now her greatest prayer has been granted by our Heavenly Father. No longer will she be frustrated by the physical limitations of her heart or her body. She can be with us twenty-four hours a day, serving, taking care of her family, ministering to people, helping them, singing to them. Serving in Joy until ...*

I started out with a strong voice, determined to finish without getting choked up or crying. My mother deserved a tribute to her life. Her friends and family needed understanding and comfort from its message. But something was happening to my voice, not because my throat was tightening with emotion. My voice sounded funny like an odd nasal sound, similar to a munchkin in "The Wizard of Oz" movie. I paused and tried to swallow, wondering if I was more emotional than I thought. But the pause did not help. It was as if my mouth could not form words.

The memorial services were completed, but there were many more people to notify, the coroner to deal with, her personal belongings, bills, business aspects and estate issues to deal with. It was the years before Internet access was available. All the death related business had to be conducted fron a wheelchair with no car and no ability to get to banks, businesses or stores.

Nagymama continued to hold on to her life in a Salt Lake City, Utah hospital intensive care unit. She had been transferred to the more sophisticated medical facility 150 miles away due to the severity of her injuries. I wanted desperately to be with her. The deleterious emotional and physical stress was now mounting at a tremendous rate.

On January 1, 1987, nine days after the accident, the University of Michigan Wolverines football team faced off against Arizona State in the celebrated annual Rose Bowl game. My friends, Kerry and Karen, knowing of my college football fanaticism, had gotten tickets to the Rose Bowl game. In their extraordinary effort to ease my grief, they drove from their home in Marina del Rey to my apartment in San Fernando Valley, picked up me and the wheelchair, drove to the Rose Bowl stadium in Pasadena, and fought through the throngs of nationwide fans to get me in my wheelchair to my seat—an act of heroism as any Southern Californian or any attendee of a Rose Bowl game well knows. My team did not do very well. After all of Kerry and Karen's heroics to cheer me, my beloved Wolverines lost to Arizona State, 22-15.

Lezione Uno: Coraggio, Leeza (Lesson One: Courage, Lisa)

The Wolverines were not the only ones not doing well. As a hard-core football fan I was hyper-focused on game action and tuned out frivolous chitchat. Arizona players approached the line of scrimmage. The Michigan players responded by positioning themselves facemask-to-facemask with their opponents. Some hit the three-point stance as the play was set. Tension in the stands was high. Suddenly the white yard lines split into doubles right before me! I blinked hard and the double lines merged back into one white line.

Okay. That was weird. Seconds later the lines split into two again. I blinked hard but this time my vision did not recover. I closed my eyelids for a few seconds but when I opened them two lines appeared where I intellectually knew there was only supposed to be one. I shifted focus from the lines to the players. What I saw was a twin of each player to his right side.

Karen was a phenomenal cardiac care unit nurse. I wanted to tell her about the double vision I just had, especially because it would not resolve. *Nah. Don't worry Karen. The double vision is just a temporary fluke. You've been under tremendous stress the past ten days. That's all it is.*

But the truth was I knew something serious and bad was happening to my body, neurologically. At the same time, it was unfathomable to think that another tragedy could occur. I was embarrassed to tell anyone of my suspicions of a neurological breakdown.

First you tell them you have rheumatoid arthritis, then you explain you can't walk any more and will miss medical school entry for that year, then you remain in a wheelchair for another year, then your mother gets killed in a car accident and your grandmother is struggling for her life in an intensive care unit. You cannot mention you are having neurological symptoms. They'll think you are a paranoid hypochondriac becoming delusional.

Rather than tell anyone what was happening I began to make excuses. A pre-med friend who had made it to medical school called me. She had caught the fact that my speech was slurred. I told her that it was only garbled because I had spent an inordinate amount of time talking on the phone counseling people grieving at the news of my mother's death or being consoled. I had told the story dozens of times over about how "My mom wanted to be in the heavenly Christmas choir and there she had her place among the angelic beings and choir loft as the Christmas dawn shown its first pink light."

"Oh that is ridiculous. You can't get slurred speech from talking too much." my school friend ridiculed.

I knew that speech does not slur from too much talking. I had studied physiology. I also knew that her superior IQ far surpassed mine and she would most likely call me out on this one. So I blew off the comment by laughing at her chiding and changed the subject.

But it was more difficult to disregard her comment in my own mind. I was now trying to convince myself I was not embarking on a scary trip toward a serious neurological disease. Rheumatoid arthritis did its best to deteriorate joints, but as long as you took precaution to avoid fatal GI bleeds or damage to heart tissue, it was not imminently fatal. Diseases such as ALS (Lou Gehrig's), Parkinson's or multiple sclerosis, with their progressive muscle degeneration, could lead to an untimely death. *There is no way God would allow me to have a neuromuscular disease on top of being crippled by rheumatoid arthritis and oppressive grief.*

The truth was I had experienced more traumatic events in a few recent months than most people experience in their entire lifetime.

Nagymama had died after a month of fighting courageously against traumatic injury and ferocious infection. Shortly before she died I had flown with my wheelchair to be at her hospital bedside. My guts wrenched to see her elegant, lengthy, supine and pain-wracked body rigid against the hospital bed. The ventilator tube was taped against the sides of her mouth, her skin an odd shade of yellow.

Nagymama, you are an incredibly generous being. You are a remarkable woman. She had been extraordinarily thoughtful and kind to others, loving and smart with a compulsion to be helpful. During World War II her life had been difficult. But after the war she made a good life out of all of the hardships with her dear husband always at her side. After all the two had bravely and victoriously endured together on both continents it was not easy to lose her beloved in the end to cancer.

Oh my dear, regal, generous Nagymama, what can I do to help you survive … to ease your pain … to infuse you with strength?

I pressed Nagymama's favorite Rosary beads into her hand and started reciting the Rosary. Nagymama was ever faithful to a daily recitation of the lovely devotional prayer. I spoke for her now those simple, beautiful, comforting, powerful words with the fervor of one whose heart was breaking, who implored God from the depths of her soul to spare this mangled and struggling woman from suffering and death; to keep her alive so at least two of my three-member California-based family could remain on this earth to physically hold one another through the grief of losing Mom-Julia.

I barely made it into the first decade of the Rosary when the prayer became choked by my contracting larynx. I broke into unleashed sobbing, pleading with her to live, gravely promising her I would take care of her.

"Oh Nagymama … please Nagymama … you've got to live… you just have to live! You are so strong … you have survived incredible tragedies … You can survive this, too. Please Nagymama, I promise you. I will make myself walk again and get a job, and support you. You have unselfishly helped care for me these past two years. I will take care of you. I will nurse you back to health. Please. Just please pull through this and come back with me to our apartment."

I saw her eyelids lift and then close. She was fighting to keep them open so as to focus on me. Even in the few minutes her eyes were partially open I could see they were bloodshot and tinged an evil yellow color. She had awakened at hearing me speak the words of her beloved Rosary and forced herself to consciousness at the call of my sobs. Recognizing me now she tried to speak, her words choked by the hard ventilator tube in her throat. Her face grimaced at the spasms of her throat against the breathing tube.

Oh no. Are you too sobbing? But it can hurt you to sob with that hard tube in your throat!

I scooted my wheelchair with my feet so I was closer to the head of the hospital bed, leaned forward to place my hand on her forehead and stroked her brow, moving down to gently touch her cheeks and smooth the gripping medical tape surrounding her mouth. She stared directly at me with large, fear-opened eyes, the only manner in which she could communicate with me at the moment. I swore she was begging, frantically pleading with me to tell her whether her beloved, bubbly, blond-ringlets adorned daughter was alive. Her lips formed around the ventilator tube and formed the word "Julia."

She tried again to ask but no sound emitted and the rigid tube rebelled against her throat and larynx. She again choked, tears streaming out of both of her frightened eyes. I knew at that moment she knew Julia was dead. I wanted so desperately to protect her from that fact, especially now when she was fighting with every ounce of being she possessed at this precarious edge. I was afraid that if she learned that her precious daughter had died, she would lose her will to live.

True to the generous reputation of Salt Lake City folk, a local family I had never known and who had never known me, opened their home to me that night. I had no job, no money to stay in a hotel or no money to offer them. Can you imagine the incredible trust and remarkable kindness it took to leave a front door open for a stranger and her wheelchair as she came and went from the hospital? One of the hospital staff had called around to friends that lived close enough to the hospital for me to travel in wheelchair.

A family had opened their home and all their possessions to me, for nothing in return. They respected my need for privacy and left the front door open and a room cleared for me to sleep; no questions asked about my situation, no questions asked about when I might be arriving or leaving. Would I ever do the same for a stranger? Their extraordinary hospitality deeply moved me but could not comfort my heart which was back in that ICU room, ripped out and bleeding on the floor. So it was not too hard to understand how I could deceive myself about an inner brewing, life-threatening neurological disease.

These were heart-wrenching times. I had learned details of the accident. It had occurred at 10:36 a.m. about fifteen miles south of the rural town of Kanosh, Utah. It was a bucolic setting—a lone stretch of highway with lush green, tree dense mountains of Fish Lake National Forest viewable on the right as the jam-packed Subaru four-wheel-drive hatch-back headed north. Evidence at the scene told that the car had veered toward the right shoulder, then jerked suddenly back on to the road. The sharp turn caused the car to flip. In the forceful momentum my mother's body was thrown from the driver seat, propelled mid-air across the highway median and landed in a fatal crushing blow on the opposite shoulder of oncoming lanes. Nagymama mercilessly tumbled about inside the car as it rolled several more times in the median.

The accident report stated: "Driver apparently fell asleep at the wheel." I was outraged! *No! There was no way my mother and grandmother's life could have ended by something as mundane and preventable as falling asleep at the wheel*! It had been a frosty morning and that stretch of Utah highway was known for its black ice. *Could the car have hit a patch of the hidden dangerous ice and Mom lost control? Perhaps Mom had reached behind her for her thermos. How dare the investigators speculate that she fell asleep! And what about her safety belt? Why had she been thrown from the car?* She always wore her safety belt, and especially on this long trek she would have kept it fastened.

There was a class action lawsuit against Subaru at the time for safety belts that would release upon impact. She would have lived if her safety belt would have held.

The emotional stress was multiplying and adding to the physical stress: I made arrangements for the cremation of my mother's body in Utah and shipment of her ashes back to me. I handled her estate issues and accompanying intense interactions with family, companies and courts. I contended with Nagymama's medical bills, sorting, calling, resolving.

With my only two personal caregivers unexpectedly dead, I did not have access to a glass for water or a bowl for food, the cupboard being too high to reach from my wheelchair. I could not afford the rent for the lovely three-room Woodland Hills apartment and would have to move. But first, I would have to sort through three generations of women's stuff. How could I do this, not being able to stand or to walk? I couldn't even propel myself over the floor molding of the apartment door to gain access to the outside world. So, with all I was directly dealing, it was not difficult to deny that my peripheral nervous system was going haywire. I could easily rationalize the abnormal physical occurrences by blaming it on extraordinary stress.

The facial muscle fatigue quickly progressed from slurred speech to having difficulty chewing and swallowing. I tried to get nourishment by drinking blended fruit shakes and protein drinks. At times even attempts to swallow thick liquids were not successful, the liquid making a dribbling escape from flaccidly loose lips. I hid the difficulty as I was embarrassed enough that

Lezione Uno: Coraggio, Leeza (Lesson One: Courage, Lisa)

I needed to use a wheelchair and I didn't want to appear as a hypochondriac. Besides, I had a few good days, especially in the mornings, where the facial muscles were not as uncooperative.

To divert from the overwhelming stress and grief, my Aunt Anne registered me in one of the infamously heralded Los Angeles offering: a one-day motivational conference. True to its advertised purpose, the workshop was motivating with a lot of interaction among the speakers or participants. A bonus was that seated next to me was a handsome Italian-American man. There were several breakout sessions to be worked on in pairs and I was delighted to be paired each time with, you guessed it, the good-looking Italian-American man. It seemed my fortune was finally turning toward the better. Not only was he an Italian Adonis, he was witty, remarkably articulate and earnestly kind. He graciously paid no heed to the fact I was seated in a wheelchair, bereft of an inability to walk or propel myself. Through the course of the day we discovered similarities in addition to Italian descent and the pronunciation of our surnames.

I was pleasantly shocked when Joseph called the following week and asked if I would have lunch with him. After all, he was an attractive, smart, spiritually-centered man, close to me in age, trying to make it in L.A. as a sports broadcaster. I felt I was just a woman in a wheelchair, trying to find my way to the surface of a world turned upside down.

Even though we were just friends, I wanted to look my best. Primping for the lunch date, I lifted my arm, as I had done thousands of times in the past, to apply mascara to my long Italian eyelashes. *Boy this arm feels heavy. Maybe it is weak?* I was seated in the wheelchair looking into a portable mirror on a pedestal. The mirror was almost the same height as my face; I barely needed to lift my arm to reach the eyelashes. I grabbed my right elbow with my left hand to act as a supportive brace. *Man, your arm feels as if it weighs a ton! Is the strength leaving because you are nervous about having lunch with a handsome man?*

I struggled with cosmetics but by the time it came to lift the curling iron it felt as if my arm had turned into a solid lead weight. I could not force my arm to budge, not with all my mind and willpower. The arm lay limp and heavy at my side. *C'mon Lisa! Concentrate. Focus on commanding your arm to move and it will!* Yet no matter how hard I tried to concentrate with my mind to force the arm to move it remained motionless and limp at my side. *Surely the arm muscle weakness was merely another result of stress.*

I decided to give up on the coifing and rest for the few minutes before Broadcaster Joseph arrived to load me and my wheelchair.

Our lunch destination was a cute outdoor café on a perfect sunny San Fernando Valley day. *Perfect also, because the menu was likely to have lighter Valley Girl fare, most likely something I am able to chew and swallow.*

As we looked over the lunch menu I remarked to Joseph, "Oh, they have fruit and yogurt smoothies. I love fruit and yogurt smoothies! I will order the peach yogurt smoothie."

I protested against his suggestions to add a salad or entrée.

We laughed and exchanged stories. The number of childhood experiences and present day philosophies we had in common was incredible. As the mood was positive, so I expected my body to be contentedly cooperative.

His entree was served. The peach smoothie, in an ornate soda-fountain glass with inserted straw, was placed in front of me. As good of an actress as I was becoming, I could not hide what would come. From the combination of laughing, talking and trying to eat, my facial muscles simply pooped out. None of the muscles of the cheeks or lips functioned well enough to pucker with enough suction to pull liquid up the straw. With exaggerated facial movement I created enough vacuum for a couple ounces of smoothie to move up the straw and into my mouth.

Lezione Uno: Coraggio, Leeza (Lesson One: Courage, Lisa)

I saw it first in the look on Joseph's face. He stopped talking mid-sentence and stared at my chin. Then I felt it. Cool liquid streaming down my chin. Tiny droplets sprayed onto my hand as the smoothie stream hit the table. I saw the little pool of peachy-pink cream. My hand flung to my chin in disbelief but sure enough it met a sticky, slippery mess. *Nooooooooo! Oh please nooooooooo!*

Instead of being swallowed, the few ounces of drink had slipped out of the limply drooping lips and dripped down my chin. The drool had not occurred alone in the privacy of my home. I had dribbled right in front of handsome him and he had noticed!

Joseph was stunned and had stopped talking, not knowing what to say. Worse yet, the nightmare hadn't ended with the inability to sip and swallow. My speech began to sound as if the smoothie drink had been spiked with alcohol. I was slurring words as if drunk. I was horrifyingly embarrassed. Joseph was incredibly gracious and understanding.

The humiliation from that incident served as impetus to face reality; go to my rheumatologist and fess up. When she walked into the exam room I apologized for suggesting I might have another serious disease. I told her my symptoms and gave her my self-diagnosis. She told me she thought I was right. She thought it prudent to rule out other potential causes of muscle weakness—multiple sclerosis or ALS.

Several vials of blood were drawn from my arm that day. She called me with the blood test results to let me know we were both correct, I had myasthenia gravis.

Biochemistry being one of my favorite subjects, I read any biochemistry-related document I discovered. I had come across the little-known neuromuscular disease myasthenia gravis during my studies. From my cursory Latin I deduced the medical term meant "heavy feeling muscles." I recalled seeing a magazine photo showing the beautiful Jackie Kennedy-Onassis with

Aristotle Onassis, his eyelids pulled open by application of transparent tape from the lid to the brow. Although Onassis had amassed enough wealth to afford any desire, not enough was known at that time of the biochemical and physiological origins of myasthenia gravis to effectively treat and prevent death. Despite affluence that could buy an entire neuromuscular research facility, Aristotle Onassis died of myasthenia gravis in Paris on March 15, 1975. For this reason perhaps, myasthenia gravis had earned a retrievable folder in my memory banks.

At the time of his death, the Muscular Dystrophy Association was conducting snake venom research. Ordinarily, the muscle of a healthy person "moves" when the nerve sends a chemical message to the muscle. Message receptor sites lie along the outer layer of muscle. The receptor site "receives" the chemical messenger sent from the nerve and thus tells it to "move."

Snake venom is neurotoxic. When a snake bites its victim, it injects neurotoxic venom. The venom blocks the nerve messenger from being received by the muscle receptor. Because the muscle cannot move if the transmission is blocked, the snake's victim experiences numbness and paralysis, which leads to respiratory failure and death.

I use two analogies to help myself visualize the neuromuscular process. In the first analogy, that of the healthy person nerve-to-muscle interaction, Mr. Nerve has a critical message it must urgently get to the action committee at their nearby headquarters. Mr. Nerve sends his critical message in a small red coupe convertible. The doorman of the prestigious Manhattan Street headquarter office building awaits the message by the parking spot designated solely for the red convertible messenger. The red convertible pulls into the parking spot and the doorman receives the message, dashes to the action committee meeting room where the message is immediately acted upon. In the second analogy, myasthenia gravis nerve-to-muscle interaction, Mr. Nerve again sends his critical message in a small red coupe convertible. But alas, evil Mr. Venom seeks to thwart the delivery of the critical message. Mr. Venom sends an imposter red convertible. The imposter convertible is about the same size as the true messenger car so it is able to pull into the parking spot. The color is recognized by the doorman so he does not prevent it from parking. Too late, as the doorman realizes it is an imposter, but there is nothing he can do. The true messenger pulls up but the parking spot is blocked. The doorman cannot receive the critical message and the action committee is prevented from carrying out the urgent instructions.

The milestone snake venom studies of the early 1970s focused on the nerve chemical messenger "acetylcholine" and accordingly the muscle receiver "acetylcholine receptor." When snake venom was used with myasthenia gravis patients it bound to the acetylcholine receptor on the muscle. The binding was expected, acting similar to the paralyzing effects of venom on other humans and animals. But what was not expected was the finding that myasthenia gravis patients had less acetylcholine receptors than healthy people. The snake venom experiment discovery led to the knowledge that the body of a myasthenia gravis patient produces antibodies to its own acetylcholine receptors. The antibodies act in an imposter manner similar to snake venom. The "real" nerve messenger acetylcholine is blocked from being received by the muscle receptor because an imposter is stuck in its parking spot.

The cure for myasthenia gravis is yet to be found. But assisted by the discovery of the corrupt acetylcholine receptor antibodies, medical scientists developed a medication that would allow for the real acetylcholine messenger to hang around the neuromuscular area in case one of the parking spots should become open for it to park. The impossibly long medical term for the medication is "anti-acetylcholine-esterase." I know it by the name on the prescription bottle, "Mestinon", or the generic chemical name "pyridostigmine bromide." It is the same drug that was carried by

U.S. soldiers during Desert Storm, to be taken in the event of a nerve gas attack.

Even though blood tests told of my myasthenia gravis diagnosis, it was confirmed by Electro-myograph (EMG) and nerve conduction tests. A needle was inserted into various muscles in my body and a series of electric shocks implemented. The results immediately and unequivocally demonstrated I had myasthenia gravis; the muscle reaction showed weakening as the electrical current pulse was repeated. Tensilon was injected into my arm and the muscle regained normal movement. It was confirmed: I had a severe onset of the neuromuscular disease myasthenia gravis.

I was started on a modest amount of Mestinon and a whopping dose of steroids. Although the steroids had a forceful negative effect on my mood, appetite, weight and sleep, it had no beneficial effect on the myasthenia gravis. The dose of Mestinon was increased, but did not bring my symptoms under control. Myasthenia gravis becomes fatal when it paralyzes the muscles that help you breathe. Danger may also come if you cannot swallow, choke, aspirate fluids into your lungs and are unable to cough up the fluids to clear the lungs. Because my facial and throat muscles remained weak, more dramatic efforts needed to be taken to bring the disease under control before my respiratory muscles pooped out, mandating intubation and reliance on a ventilator to breathe.

In 1987, Intravenous Immunoglobulin (IVIG) treatment for myasthenia gravis was not readily available to me. Some myasthenia gravis patients experienced remission when their thymus glands were surgically removed. My thymus gland did not appear enlarged and I was not physically stable enough to undergo surgery, so the thymectomy option was excluded.

Plasma pheresis was reserved for patients in myasthenic crisis. At that moment I was in a myasthenic crisis. Plasma pheresis, as it was explained to me, was a type of blood dialysis. Blood from my body would be taken from a vein in one arm and run through a dialysis machine, similar to the blood filtering process in kidney dialysis. In kidney dialysis body waste and impurities were the target to be filtered out of whole blood and discarded, substituting for the cleansing function of the kidney. In plasma pheresis the target was antibodies, antibodies found in the translucent, yellowish plasma portion of whole blood. The goal of plasma pheresis was for the dialysis machine to capture and filter the larger white blood cells from the plasma portion of my blood and to return as much of the antibody-free plasma and red blood cells as possible.

Antibodies are included in the bastion of white blood cells. In most instances, antibodies are good soldiers, attacking any foreign entities that may enter the human body. The opposite is true in myasthenia gravis and other autoimmune diseases where the body produces antibodies that attack or fight against itself, thus the term "auto-immune."

My body produced imposter antibodies that blocked the acetylcholine receptors on my muscle tissues. The nerve messenger being blocked from the receptor on my muscle meant that particular muscle was prevented from moving; not good when I needed muscle to swallow or breathe. Thus, plasma pheresis dialysis was employed to extract whole (heterogenous) blood, use centrifugal force to separate the antibody components from the red blood cells, and discard the entire congregation of antibodies. The hope with plasma pheresis was that by throwing away all the antibodies, enough of the muscle receptor imposter antibodies would be absent to enable the acetylcholine messenger to find an unobstructed muscle receptor, park, and entice a muscle to contract.

To a biochemist such as me who believed I was living in the scientifically advanced age of the 1980s, the procedure sounded archaic. *Hey, why not perform a non-specific invasive procedure in hopes of throwing out a little bad with a lot of good. Why discriminate* against the good cells? What did they ever do wrong to deserve to be trashed? Isn't that throwing out the baby with the bath water? And don't I need a significant level of antibodies to fight off viruses, bacteria and other foreign invaders? While I might be ridding my blood of receptor-blocking imposter antibodies, aren't I also leaving my body defenseless against infectious disease and malevolent cells?*

There were no finer options offered. I was desperate. I could no longer eat or speak clearly, and coupled with fear from my doctor that the muscle weakness would spread to swallowing and breathing, I eagerly agreed to a course of plasma pheresis treatment.

Adding to the complexity of the procedure was the fact that I could not walk, much less drive. In this exacerbated state of myasthenia gravis I needed the several hours-long plasma pheresis procedure three times a week. Being in a wheelchair for the past two years I no longer owned a car. *How was I going to drive myself from my apartment in the San Fernando Valley to the hospital in North Hollywood-Burbank where I would get the treatment? Your caregiver-driver-mother has just been killed in a car accident. The remaining members of your family live almost a continent away. All of your California college friends have commenced their new careers in full-time jobs. Plasma pheresis is a must if you want to survive. But how? Dear God, please help me figure out a way ...*

These were the circumstances that led to my residence in the nursing home located close to the apheresis-capable hospital. From that nursing home setting a nurse aide would fetch me in the quiet early morning hours, swing me from the edge of my hospital bed into my wheelchair, and push me to the facility's entrance door. I would wait at that entrance, at least three times a week, for the medical transport van. Loaded and strapped down, the van driver would shuttle me to the hospital's entrance where again I would wait, my arms too pain-frozen from rheumatoid arthritis and too weak from myasthenia gravis to propel my manual wheelchair. A hospital transport person would whisk me through the hospital to the room where the apheresis machine sat waiting to suck blood from its next sufferer. The transport man or woman would patiently and cautiously transfer my body from the wheelchair into a bed that was aligned parallel to the dialysis machine. From that point forward an incredibly sympathetic and competent apheresis nurse would take charge.

Phew! I am already exhausted! It is not even 8:30 a.m., the procedure has not even begun, but the effort it has taken to get dressed, wait and be transported has drained me of the energy charge for the day.

I laid back and tried to relax, believing a centered state of mind would ease the needle insertion phase. A large needle needed to be inserted into the vessel of one arm to draw my blood into the apheresis machine. Another large needle was inserted into the opposite arm in order to return the blood that had been stripped of antibodies. The diameter of both the ingoing and outgoing needles needed to be wide in order to avoid damage to the red blood corpuscles that would be extracted and hopefully returned to my circulatory system. The needle was not only wide, it appeared to be two inches of cold, rigid metal. Insertion of the seeming inflexible, large pipe into the slippery vessel of a debilitated patient was a sweat-inducing feat of luck for even the most skilled of technicians. Due to the width of the needle and the length that needed to be threaded up the vessel, it rarely was. Either the needle would puncture or slice through the vessel, or burst from the blood flow pressure, or the vessel would poop out and collapse minutes or hours into the procedure. At times a beautiful, engorged vessel would appear after the tourniquet was applied. The hopeful prospect of the seemingly easy pipeline could be dashed if the vessel would roll out of reach after the needle punctured the skin. The options and success rate diminished with the number of prior insertions. The threat of implanting a central venous line, either in the jugular, subclavian or groin area grew heavier with each insertion failure.

The apheresis nurse scrubbed a potential insertion site on each arm with smelly, brown-staining Betadyne antiseptic; she scrubbed the skin hard and long and I could feel my deteriorated elbows crack in and out of place with her force.

The nurse seems as anxious as you about a successful insertion of the harpoons. You need to pray. Just lay back your head and pray. Dear Lord, please send the Holy Spirit to infuse this nurse with the confidence, wisdom and peace she needs for successful insertion. Please, dear Lord, make the first go-around be successful and have it remain prosperous throughout the entire several-hour procedure.

"Okay Lisa, it is going to take me several seconds after you feel the needle poke to thread the needle into the vein. I need you to lie very still until I tell you that you can move. Can you do that for me?"

"Mmm-hmm." I already had my head pushed back into the pillow and my lips tightened; anticipating what was soon to come.

"It helps to take a long, slow breath, making a sucking sound for the length of the time I am inserting the needle. Are you ready? Go."

I made a small round hole with my lips and started noisily sucking air into my lungs. I forced my mind to picture myself standing in a sun-drenched meadow, waist high in plentiful yellow and white daisies. I applied other senses and went further into the picture; feeling the warmth of the sun on my face, feeling the emotions of happy and content as yellow and white happy faces danced around me …

Arrghhh! It hurts! I screamed and shook with pain in my mind, not daring to move my physical body as I felt wet sweat form on my forehead.

After a couple of agonizing passes I had an extraction and a return line in place. Only a modest amount of blood could be outside of my body at a time to prevent any blood pressure drop problems. Coupled with the unsophistication of the apheresis machines used on me in the 1980s, the pheresis procedure took several hours.

Typically I did not return to the nursing home until after 3:30 p.m. During those long hours I could not read. I was paranoid to move my arms, much less hold a book for fear a vessel would blow, necessitating a halt in the procedure while a new painful needle insertion was attempted. I stopped my mind from inquiring whether my bladder was full; the horrendous hassle and time it would take to unhook and rehook for a potty break was unfathomable. I pretty much laid there with my arms outstretched, palms facing up, hour after long hour.

It gave me reassurance that St. Joseph's was a Catholic hospital. In the apheresis room a Crucifix hung on the wall directly in front of me. As I lay there staring at it hour after hour, an elucidation came. There was symmetry between that Holy Crucifix and me—His arms outstretched and punctured with spikes; my arms outstretched and punctured with needle spikes; Him looking at me; me looking at Him. Those long hours were unspeakable theological reflections on His suffering and spiritual revelation on my suffering. Those hours of Crucifix reflection brought about an otherwise unattainable spiritual strengthening and reassurance, and in the important preoccupation, the hours passed more quickly in that strident effort.

At times I would make conversation with the apheresis nurse, but I did not want to distract her from her duties. Sometimes I would close my eyes and hope to doze off. The apheresis procedure drained me of energy as it drained my blood and I felt wiped-out tired. But I was afraid to close my eyes unless I was assured sleep would come immediately. I did not want to be left conscious with the images of the last couple of months played upon the screens of my closed eyelids.

Upon completion of the pheresis, I again sucked in my breath as the needles were painfully pulled from my aching arms. Pressure bandages were immediately applied to the insertion sites to stop any profuse and prolonged bleeding. Although my arms were sore, the pressure felt good.

After enough time passed to ensure my blood pressure was stable I was loaded back into the transport van for delivery to the nursing home. Using the handles on the back of my wheelchair a nurse aide would roll me to my destination.

My room being the furthest from the entrance, the full length of the hall had to be traversed. I uncharacteristically hung my head and stared at the carpet to avoid eye contact with my co-inhabitants and I came to know the location, circumference and color of each stain along that runway.

Courage is:

- Having faith when you are faced with the impossible.
- Moving forward even when you are faced with the impossible.
- Living again even though the ones you love most are no longer living.
- Researching the origins of and treatment options for an illness.

CHAPTER 8

In the Depths of the Soul's Dark Night

AT LEAST THE ADMINISTRATORS OF THE NURSING HOME WERE KIND ENOUGH to place me in a room with the resident closest to me in age. I had recently turned 26 years old; she was in her early 30s. From the looks of the residents parked in the hall, everyone else had us beat by about 50 years. It might have been a lifesaver to converse with my roommate, therefore keeping my mind from lurking dark thoughts. Yet the lack of oxygen to her brain during a diving accident had destroyed her cognitive ability to carry on a conversation with me.

At various times of the day or night I witnessed her open her eyes wide, lift her head slightly off the pillow and look around the room. *I wonder if she can see.* I recalled from my recent pre-med classes that at least her brain stem had function in order for her heart to be beating and for her to be breathing on her own. But it seemed to me that a lot more of her brain than just the stem was functioning for her to seem alert and looking around. *What part of her brain, if any, was processing incoming stimuli? And if info was incoming, what does she perceive?*

There was a sink and mirror on the wall facing each of our beds. If I looked straight ahead I could see my reflection in the mirror. If I looked at an angle I could see my roommate's reflection. I do not recall ever leaving my room for a meal. I do not recall ever leaving my room for a non-medical procedure except for the time Ruth brought me to Mass or Patti and Neal snuck me out the back door to the corner pub. There was no phone in the room and I do not recall a television or radio, or I might not have been able to afford their services. My environment being thus devoid of entertaining diversion, I spent a lot of time in my nursing home bed working desperately to keep positive thoughts playing in my mind and working just as desperately to keep the recent circumstances leading to my present home as far from my consciousness as possible. I lay still, hospital bed slightly inclined, trying not to disturb my body, my arms throbbing from pheresis, joints screaming from rheumatoid arthritis. When I opened my eyes from that position I tried not to focus on the mirror in my line of vision.

At times when my glance met the mirror, my roommate was staring into the mirror looking directly at me. Her stare directly bore into me, eyes unblinking. *Ooooo … that is too eerie. I am all by myself at the end of this hall. She is supposed to be in a coma. I don't understand this semi-conscious state and it is freaking me out!* I felt the hairs rise on my arms and I fought an oncoming feeling of fright.

Lezione Uno: Coraggio, Leeza (Lesson One: Courage, Lisa)

After several days and trying to figure out the origin of my fright of being left alone with a supposed comatose but contrarily semi-conscious being, I decided the compassionate thing to do was to talk with her. She was a sweet woman, who, much like me, did not choose her lot in life to include a stay in this skilled nursing facility. So when it appeared she was in the awakened state of her semi-conscious condition, I told her my name and thanked her for sharing her room with me. I told her I had seen her children and they were very cute and she should be proud they were well-mannered. I told her what day it was and what the weather conditions were for that day. I complained about how long it took for the nursing staff to respond to my call button and how awful the globs of mush meal tasted. To the last statement I thought it best not to complain about food to her, as I had never seen her eat solid food; she merely subsided on canned liquid drained down a tube into her gut. To all my chatter she never responded, but I believed that on the chance that she perceived conversation at any level, it would be stimulating and heart-warming to provide verbal human contact.

I am not sure if it was because I could not walk and the nursing facility was concerned about liability if I fell transferring myself out of bed into my wheelchair and from my wheelchair onto the toilet, but I was not allowed to use the bathroom without assistance. The nurse aides may have perceived it took too much of their time to help me into and out of the bathroom because they rarely allowed me the privilege of privacy in a bathroom, but instead insisted I use a bedpan. Have you ever tried to have a bowel movement perched on the edge of a cold, hard plastic bedpan, lying flat on your back in bed with the door open for all hallway passersby to view? And if you somehow managed to be successful in that compromising condition, have you ever had to lay in the warm putrid mess for a long period of time, gagging at the smell and being horrified by the knowledge that other occupants of your room are gagging on the odor of your fecal creation?

I promise ... when I become a doctor I will work for a federal health facility regulation that mandates a person be assisted to the privacy of a bathroom instead of left to evacuate bladder and bowel into a bedpan or diaper for the convenience of the nurse aide staff.

When I had the urge to relieve myself of bladder or bowel I looked around in panic for my call button. *Please God make the call button be within reach so that I can summon an aide for the bedpan.* No matter how many times I begged, in both English and Spanish, no matter how alert I tried to be to the location of the call button, inevitably when a nurse aide would come into the room to check vitals, or the cleaning person came into the room to sweep, or the meal tray server came into the room to place the tray on the bedside table, the call button would be moved to a location outside of my reach. The lifeline-relocating-perpetrator would be out of sight and call range within seconds, leaving both me and my roommate without any means of communicating from the enclosed far end of the nursing home. Sometimes it would take a half hour for an aide to appear at my door after pressing the call button and responding to the intercom above my head that I needed to use the bathroom.

I promise ... when I become a doctor I will forge an awareness campaign to ensure all patient call buttons and light cords be left within reach as each health professional, nurse aide and cleaning staff exits the room. Perhaps I will make it a mandatory section of a medical and nursing school class, nurse aide certification, maybe even health facility accreditation rule.

On more than one occasion the registered nurse in charge of passing meds brought me incorrect medications. One nurse in particular would stand next to me and smile, motioning for me to put into my mouth the several pills in the little paper cup she handed me. I had learned to examine the pills before ingesting. I stared into the cup now and did not recognize two of the pills. My life-sustaining Mestinon, two 60-milligram tablets every three hours needed to continue breathing and swallowing, was not among them. I tried to explain that two of the medications were not mine but she did not understand English. She appeared to be of Asian heritage and I unfortunately was without knowledge of any word in any Asian language. I resorted to hand motions and mime, but I think she believed I was being obstinate and tried to force me to take the pills, including the pills that were not mine. *I wonder who got my batch of pills?*

With my deformed fingers I managed to pick up the brownish-red gel capsule, held it out and shrugged my shoulders with a quizzical look on my face. "What is this one?"

I got no answer, and instead she insisted, "Take!"

I shook my head from side to side in a mimicked "No" then repeated my question in a simple two-word sentence, "What is?"

"Stool. Everyone take. *You* take!" With her last broken order she pushed my pill-grasping fingers to my lips. My arms weak and sore, held no defense.

Oh my, this is a stool softener! An absolute no-no for me! How do I explain to her with such a huge language barrier that after several years of taking mega-doses of aspirin my gastrointestinal tract is raw and I have a serious diarrhea problem? I can't take this pill. It would be disastrous ... and with no ability to use a toilet and no one to respond quickly with a bedpan this pill is seconds from passing through my lips. What do I do?

I don't know from where the saving thought came, but I reacted instantly and sprung my fingers open. The tiny pill fell into the bed sheets. I thrashed my thighs quickly enough for the pill to fling to the ground before she could rescue it from the sheets and force it into my mouth. I was spared for the moment but what would I do next time? There were no resident phones in the rooms. *Are there no phones because the residents either have dementia ... or facial paralysis from stroke?* I had no way of contacting the nursing home administration to express concerns about my care. My wheelchair was folded and locked against the far wall, no way for me to reach it, and my legs had not carried my weight for two years. Because my room was the last at the end of a hall, there was no hall traffic of administrative staff on his or her way to any offices. *And what if you complain? Will the nurse aides retaliate for the tattle-tale? What if you have to sit in your urine and feces for hours? You have to beg as it is for a nighttime wash cloth and toothbrush. What if you never again receive them? What if your medications and stool softeners are mixed into your food without any ability to discern whether correct?* I decided to grin and bear it, remaining vigilant and advocating for my roommate and me to the best of my ability.

And advocate I did for my roommate, that dear soul without a voice to speak for her needs or in defense of her dignity. Sometime after 9 p.m., when the post-supper and bedtime business had subsided, a nurse would administer a tube feeding to my roommate. I was not exactly sure of the location, but an opening had been made somewhere in her gastrointestinal tract and a tube inserted. The tube would serve as the vehicle through which a nutrient rich formula would be poured into her esophagus, stomach or intestines. It was from this tube feeding method that my roommate would receive her nutrition and hydration.

Although tube feeding appears to be an efficient method of delivering food and nutrition, the procedure is also fraught with peril: vomiting and aspiration. My roommate was no exception to the peril of post-feeding vomiting, especially as the result of a harried nurse rushing the contents of the canned formula into her gut.

No gagging noise would sound warning; rather the splatter of viscous vomit splayed onto the floor tile and under my bed jolted me from sleep or my fervent attempt to fall asleep. The rising odor of regurgitated enteral formula reached my olfactory senses to confirm my suspicion. If by some merciful miracle my call button had not been removed from my reach I would summon a staff person and assert the need for immediate attention.

For the same reason that my roommate made no gagging sound, I recalled from my pre-med studies that the significantly damaged portions of her brain left her defenseless to cough-up vomit that may have been mistakenly inhaled into her lungs during regurgitation. If she did not receive assistance with airway clearing she risked drowning in her own vomit or aspiration pneumonia. I was unable to get out of bed and walk to help her but I could try my darndest to get someone who could help.

After attention had been given to my roommate I would plead for the vomit to be removed from our floor. At times it would be mopped away within fifteen minutes. At other times it would be several hours, perhaps the next morning before someone would mop the sickeningly smelly vomit from the floor next to and under our beds.

As the nurses, aides or housekeeping staff entered the darkened, middle of the night room, stinging, fluorescent lights would shockingly be switched on above my bed, her bed, or both our beds. I would try to stave off middle of the night fatigue in an attempt to catch the exiting staff person and request the lights be extinguished, but at least once or twice each night the piercing, buzzing, florescent lights would remain emblazoned, pull cord or switch against a distant wall and out of reach in my bed-bound condition. In such a sleep deprived and dependent situation, an inconsiderate act of leaving on bright and buzzing lights with no means by which to turn them off or beckon someone to turn them off led to further inability to sleep, further exhaustion and helpless exasperated feelings. I felt as if stranded on an island, the search boat visible on the horizon, too far away for me to signal. Bright light and loud noise sleep deprivation have been documented methods of prisoner torture. I understood that night-shift nursing staffs were preoccupied, tired and busy; but the result of seemingly inconsequential neglect of millisecond switching off lights and removal of call button was nonetheless hours-long torture for me.

Looking back a decade later on my nursing home experience I realized many of the aspects that stripped a person of their dignity were avoidable. Public awareness and institutional movement toward improving the dignity-sparing aspects have been enacted. But at the time it was a battle to remain in positive emotion. I consciously applied humor and gratitude to fight against feeling a loss of dignity. It was not an optimal situation and it took constantly employed vigilance to avoid sliding into negative thought, anxiety or depression.

It wasn't the smell of bodily fluids or excrement that most greatly distressed me. My health advocate experience in preparation for becoming a doctor working as a nurse aide in a skilled nursing facility for the Dominican Sisters fostered an acceptance of the smells or sights of fresh or putrefying body parts and fluids as a normal, realistic part of the life process. It was not the sight of my fellow residents, most perched at death's doorstep that disturbed me. I had faced the real possibility of dying during the process of being diagnosed with rheumatoid arthritis and ruling out aggressive deadly bone cancer. I was not afraid of death. I had lived my short years to the fullest, I was grateful for the richness of love and splendid experiences, and I believed there was a glorious life awaiting me after death.

The lingering ache left by harpoon-sized needles inserted day-long in both arms for myasthenia blood dialysis: *painful*. The rheumatoid arthritis, its violent assaults against all of my joints unfettered by any treatment medical science could offer: *terribly painful*. But nothing, absolutely nothing, was as painful as knowing that *she* was dead.

As evening descended upon the nursing home halls the cacophony of howling dementia call-outs would diminish to the lone and occasional crier. Staff bustle would settle. The room lights were turned out and the heavy door nearly shut. It was then *the haunting* would begin.

Lezione Uno: Coraggio, Leeza (Lesson One: Courage, Lisa)

Every muscle in my body was fatigued, all energy of spirit depleted. *It is okay tonight. You are tired. You will fall asleep and rest. Oh dear Lord in heaven … I beg of you … please help me fall asleep quickly. Grant me peace, oh Lord … Allow me rest …*

But my battered, scarred and throbbing psyche had another agenda. It had years of tumbled and unresolved resentment and hurts, solidified into repression by a flash-pan of shock and horror to chip away and sort before it could begin its healing cycle. The dark, semi-stillness of that nursing home room kick-started the nearly exploding subconscious, employing a chisel against frozen repression. As the tangled hurt, resentments, grief and guilt unraveled, the reels began to play horror film after horror film, sometimes rewinding for a rerun just as excruciating as the initial play …

Film Scene One:

I see myself parked in the wheelchair, inside the doorstep of our apartment. Already outside the doorstep, my mother is loaded with bulging purse and last load of packages to carry to the car as she departs on her trip. She leans down and forward to place a good-bye kiss on my cheek. I see her angelic face, an expression of endearing smile as she contemplates placing a gesture of affectionate good-bye on the cheek of the one she loves. Immediately prior to her kiss reaching my cheek, I turn away so that the kiss is misplaced on the callous hairs above my left ear. She lingers anyway at the place where her rejected kiss ended, her petite nose and high cheekbone tenderly resting against my skull. I feel the warm love for her daughter, I smell the sweetness of her soul, I sense the light of her aura.

I feel an actual physical stabbing pang of regret near my heart at watching that scene.

That was your very last chance to say good-bye and you blew it! It was an opportunity to finally tell her you loved her and you thwarted the last opportunity you would ever have to look her in those blue eyes and whisper into her ears the three most vital words in the universe! And you squandered both opportunities in an action that deeply hurt her feelings! Your very last seconds of contact with her on this earth, you filled with bitterness and injury. Waste and harm … all out of resentment and stupid pride!

Next film scene:

I see myself sitting in the wheelchair holding the white corded telephone to my ear, waiting to be transferred to the Utah state police trooper in possession of the purse found at the scene of the car accident. I plead with her to search for the Christmas card presented to my mother at the doorstep departure. I picture the state trooper reluctantly digging through my mother's full-size, bottomless purse, unsure of whether she will locate the letter. I recognize that throughout the scene I have withheld my breath. As if to an inanimate television screen I urge my character, *breathe … c'mon, take a breath, Lisa.* But the Lisa character in the scene continues to hold her breath. The state trooper's hand retracts from the purse with the Christmas card in hand. I see the name "Mom" written in blue felt pen-exaggerated cursive across the front of the envelope. I see the decorative blue Christmas scroll at right angles in the bottom left corner of the card's envelope. I see the trooper's hand turning the card over, slowly turning for me to view whether the seal has been broken. After ten years I had *finally* told Mom … I *had* written it … that I *loved her.*

With carefully chosen, freely poured-forth love and gratitude I told her I loved her and I was deeply thankful for all the love and help she gave me. The conveyance was a significant act on my part and as if to signify the importance I protected its privacy by sealing.

Now watching the scene play before me I clearly see the seal had not been opened. Disappointment rushes into me as quickly as the held breath escapes. The carefully placed words had not been read. The genuine feelings of love and gratitude hidden for years behind a mask of unforgiving coldness would not be recognized in her living moments on earth. The physical feeling as the sealed envelope passed before hit me with a crushing blow to the chest, the force so intense I thought the air would explode through my eardrums.

Perhaps she would have known you loved her if you would have extended your face for her to kiss. Instead you turned away. There was only one way for her to interpret your vengeful act and it was that you continued to withhold love from her. You had been too resentful, too proud, just plain stupid and gave up your last chance to tell her or to gesture that you truly did love her, that you were deeply grateful for all she had done for you. And you were unkind to Nagymama, too. She dedicated a large part of her life to care for you, to encourage you toward medical school, and yet you were sassy with her when you were in great pain; you were judgmental of her when you were frustrated with your own physical decline preventing you from entering medical school.

The reels never seemed to stop playing rerun after rerun. I mentally tried to erase the films but canned films with even darker subject matter would arise.

Next scene:

A long stretch of barren highway. A four-wheel-drive hatchback veers into the right shoulder, quickly corrects with a sharp left turn. Rebelling against the sharp change in course the car goes end-over-end across the pavement. The body of a tall blond woman ejects from a window and shoots midair with the velocity of 60-mile-an-hour speed to land beautiful face first on the gritty asphalt shoulder of the highway's opposite lanes. The car continues to flip several times in the concave medium, forcefully tumbling inside its elegant occupant. *Nooooo! Oh God no! Stop! God make it stop! Stop the image now!*

In the dark and stillness of the nursing home night these dark thoughts forced their way to the surface of my consciousness and tormented me. For years I had known about and utilized the power of positive thinking to get me through the toughest situations. I practiced biofeedback, meditation and prayer to help overcome pain and foster a centering, peace-filled inner place conducive of healing. I employed daily gratitude attitude to stay positive about being in a wheelchair instead of medical school and hopeful I would soon walk through medical school doors. But it was excruciatingly painful to live through the sudden and horrific deaths of my beloved mother and grandmother. No matter how hard I worked at changing my thoughts about their deaths to positive or peaceful, no matter how earnestly I prayed for their souls and the peace and strength to deal with loss of those monumental figures in my life, my thoughts would revert and the physical throbbing ache would return to my heart and gut. *It has to be easier to be the person who died than to live in this angst and yearning of grief.*

In those besieged moments I would desperately call forth every self-help method and every divine being I could think of to help me survive, emotionally and physically. *C'mon Lisa!* I had always been able to pull myself through the toughest adversity. But this truly was the darkest hour of my soul. I saw myself slipping down a dark, frigid, slimy tube. The creepy chilled slime prevented my hands from bracing my body against the sides of the tube. *You are slipping further down.* With all the emergency training I had I was accustomed to remaining calm through precarious traumatic situations. *Don't worry you can always pull yourself up. But where is the rope to pull yourself up and out of the black hole? How come you can't see it?*

I also had survival skills training from scout years and my outdoors-loving parents. I told myself to remain calm. *Close your eyes and use senses other than your eyes to find the lifesaving rope. Feel it within your grasp.* I had always been able to find some survival tool. *If you cannot see or feel the rope, find a crag or rock to manage a foothold.* But no matter what resource I could summon, what solution I could derive, a negative thwarted a positive outcome.

I started to panic, battling the feeling of slipping deeper into that dark hole. Maybe I would not make it this time. Maybe it was all too much.

Courage is:

- Fighting the plunge into the dark night of hopelessness, fear and depression.
- Forgiving another and expressing that forgiveness before it is too late to convey the message on earth.

CHAPTER 9

Life Lessons About Courage from Nonna

"*Coraggio, Leeza. Coraggio.*"

A soft voice, the words sounding nothing more than a wisp on the dark folds of the night.

"What?"

I heard my one-worded question echo through the sterile, tiled, darkened nursing home room. Other than me there was no person in the room capable of speaking. Yet I had heard the words …

"*Coraggio, Leeza. Coraggio.*"

The command was firm and steady now. Then silence. And in that silence the words registered.

Yes. Yes, Nonna. YES!

Tingling sensations ran through me as revelation sprung forth. Nonna had extraordinary determination coupled with determination, a positive attitude and faith that God was on her side. She did not merely talk about *coraggio*, she lived her life courageously.

I recognized her *coraggio* from the many stories she told about her first years in America. She arrived in Detroit, Michigan directly from Southern Italy. Neither she, her parents nor her siblings understood a word of English. She was of school age and entered a public school class where, not only had her classmates already spent years as friends, they had spent several years learning foundational curriculum. Her teacher was pretty and kind-mannered, but only spoke English. Her family had no money for clothes and shoes. They had never seen snow or experienced a bitter Midwest American winter.

As winter laid its blankets of snow on her path to school Nonna determinedly figured out a way to get there. A big-hearted neighbor had handed down a pair of shoes two sizes too large. She took a pair of her mother's old worn, thick, black cotton stockings and slid them in and pulled them over the clown-sized shoes. The stockings prevented the clown shoes from getting stuck in the deep snow and flipping off her feet. But worn cotton stockings did not prevent her feet from becoming bitterly cold and wet. Her teacher and classmates watched her remove the sodden worn stockings from her feet and lay them on the floor near the classroom door each day in hopes they would dry before the trek home. But the foot gear left her feet wet and cold for the remainder of the day.

Food was also scarce at home. On her walk to school one hand was warm from the night-roasted chestnut and piece of bread placed in her pocket for lunch, but the meager portion wasn't enough to keep her from being hungry.

Despite the adversities, Nonna looked forward to and attended elementary school each day, even though she knew not a word of English and had no idea what her admired teacher was saying; and she attended each day with a positive attitude. She did not focus on the fact that she was wet, cold, and hungry. She dismissed any offense from snide classmates about her mismatched clothing and peculiar lunch. It was as if her determination and elation made her oblivious to the potentially hurtful schoolmates' actions. She was in school! She was being handed an opportunity to learn and she was going to embrace every nugget of that opportunity as if is it was a chunk of precious gold.

That outlook of courage and forging ahead with a positive view was characteristic of the ways of the Old Country. In the Old Country, every spot of dirt on the steep sloping, scrappy hillside was viewed as a golden opportunity to grow food for loved ones or to produce income. The landscape into which each inhabitant was born was not viewed as a doomsday. *"There is no means to water a crop on this slope. We should not invest time in trying to farm on a slope that may erode."* No! The inhabitants of Provencia Cosenza, Italy had devised a hand-forged irrigation system using the natural slope's yield to gravity as a means of water movement. The crops themselves prevented the soil from eroding. Even the most stubborn patches of land were made fruitful by olive trees, prickly pear, fig trees, and grapevine bushes.

Courage's tunneled vision toward opportunity was Nonna's Old World psychological programming. And now, when I needed it most, I awakened to the fact that through her examples it was my psychological programming as well. All I needed was to view *my* situation through courage's tunneled vision toward opportunity.

What other aspects of courage have been shown to you? Gratitude and ingenuity.

In Nonna's Old World village each family was allowed to use the community outdoor brick oven one designated day per week.

The families did not view having to share one, non-private oven as a limitation, but rather as an appreciated aspect of the community. On day five and six, the flat round loaves of bread were not viewed as stale rocks in need of discard. No! Rich, home-pressed olive oil and savory dried oregano and basil were massaged into the hardened crust creating *focaccio*. Ingenuity and a positive view turned stale rocks into a tasty sustenance.

The survival tools born of courage became clearer to me now. *And what about love and faith? Was it faith that made courage possible? Or does it take courage to maintain faith in heart-breaking, or apparently hopeless or seemingly unjust situations?*

I recalled the tears in Nonna's eyes when she told me how she treasured going to school and learning, and how it broke her heart when in seventh grade her parents reluctantly forced her to quit. She was the oldest child, and unlike her parents, she had learned to speak English. Instead of her attending school, she was needed to work, to earn money and help support the family.

At the age of fourteen Nonna recognized love of family was paramount and forever left behind organized schooling to aid in her family's survival. With *coraggio* in hand and faith that God would provide for her, she landed a sewing job in a steaming hot pants factory; in the sweltering Detroit summers the temperature would rise to unbearable levels. But Nonna worked with gratitude, pride and diligence. Within no time she convinced the owner of the pants factory to give her extra work so her pay could be increased.

The financial needs of her family continued. With a deep inhalation of courage she again entered the office of her boss, and as a result, each night she carried home a heavy cloth sack of unfinished pants. After dinner, no matter how exhausted they all were, she, her mother, and her father, sat together in the front room and finished stitching the entire lot of pants. The following morning, Nonna would return the bundles and receive a few cents for each pair of pants that were hand-finished. Yet, still her weekly income, including pay for the extra work and take-home sewing, was sparse. In addition, in order to reach the pants factory she had to walk a great distance carrying the heavy bundle of take-home pants and pay a nickel each way for the streetcar.

On her way to the streetcar, Nonna would look up at the placard of a pickle factory. *Now who wouldn't find advertisement of a pickle factory peculiarly interesting?* One night, exhaustedly drudging home, struggling with the unmanageable sack of pants pieces, she stopped in front of the pickle factory. She dropped the sack to the ground. Armed with courage and faith she marched into the pickle factory and found her way to the owner. With a deep breath she stood before him and asked for a job. The owner did not respond. He looked at her from head to toe. Here was a woman off the street in terribly matched clothes, firmly requesting a job after 6 p.m.

"I wouldn't leave and he didn't know what to say," Nonna explained to us decades later.

But she stood firm in her courage and faith.

"I am very strong and I promise I will work very hard for you," she told the owner of the pickle factory.

The owner hesitated again, but within a few minutes she had a new job in the pickle factory.

She worked diligently and loyally.

"I was the fastest pickle packer at one point," Nonna told us proudly. "And I lifted those heavy crates of packed quart jars better than some men!"

She gained the respect of the owner and the foremen. It was not just a pickle packing job to her. She had stepped out in faith; the owner had taken a chance on her and she would not disappoint him.

When Nonna became pregnant with my father, the pickle factory owner assured her it was okay to take time off before the birth. Still determined, she worked as close to the day she would give birth to her first *figlio* (son) as the owner allowed, then returned to work soon after her son was born.

Decades later I witnessed Nonna's courage and faith after my *Nonno* (grandfather) Francesco died. Back in the 1930s thru 1950s, an Italian-American wife did not learn to drive nor learn household finances. The Italian wife was backdrop to her husband's center stage performance. So after my Nonno died, we worried what would come of Nonna. How would she survive? Again, Nonna's courage, faith, and unquestioning belief trusted that God would take care of her even though her husband, provider and best friend was gone.

Nonna's soul-certainty was so absolute it never occurred to her that God might not take care of her. Her courageous reliance on the benevolence of God avoided any attitude of pity and dependence. Although her gregarious husband may have commanded the household and family during their long marriage, she had a clean canvas with which she could paint a life that would harvest joy and fulfillment. Although already well into her sixties, I watched her create a new, independent life by leaning on nothing more than courage, faith and determination.

Her words of advice had well-earned credibility: "Fight and don't ever give up, *Leeza*", she encouraged me. "You do whatever you believe is right for *you* and do not listen to anybody else," she would often repeat.

In the past I had battled and moved forward using that encouragement and support, and it all stemmed from Nonna's *primo principale* (prime principle): *corrrr-a-jeee-o* (courage).

Courage never failed Nonna and it's power afforded her extraordinary feats. Now, lying in the middle of the night in a nursing home bed, I was in the most crucial battle of my life, through the darkest and longest night of my life.

People more learned, wise, and holier than me have taught that it is in the darkest hour of the soul that a flicker of light can be seen—a light that becomes brighter as the soul searches for

the origin of that light; a light that becomes illuminating as the
soul is drawn toward it in a desperate effort to be drawn out of
a eagerly swallowing vortex of blackened quicksand; and it is in
the illuminating light that the soul recognizes a path. The light
may not reveal the entire path or the magnificent kingdom to
which the path leads. But even a mere spark-sized illuminating
of the soul may give just enough radiance to guide it in the right
direction.

The illuminated guidance transforms souls and rearranges
thoughts. But it isn't until a person reaches the darkest, most desperate moment that a flicker of light can be noticed or given the
undivided attention it takes to guide us to transformation. A person may not gain an understanding of why their loved one was
senselessly murdered or taken from them in a fatal car accident,
or suffered a long, painful, degenerative disease; but through the
dark night process they know what they must do with that experience. Yes, a person is left with the fact that the murder, the fatal
car accident, or the prolonged disease occurred. But nothing can
erase that misfortunate occurrence. The person can see where
they need to move from that moment forward. The movement
may be to change a part of them that was dying due to resentment, hatred or harmful habits. The movement may be to incul-
cate a unique empathy with which to reach out to others who are
soon to experience unjust, illogical or painful occurrences.

For me, in that dark nursing home night, the illuminating
light appeared in the form of a faint whisper from a dim and cob-
webbed corner of my mind. I had heard whispered recollections
of encouragement bestowed years past by a wise and concerned
grandmother. In the tone of her expression and in the look of
knowledge born through trial I realized that her belief in and in-
sistence on *coraggio* came as a result of not one, but several dark
nights of her own soul.

In my darkened, enclosed nursing home room that night,
senses devoid of any light or sound to distract, I reflected on the

challenges of Nonna's life and how her reliance on *coraggio* enabled her to take a step forward to act, and with that action good would happen in her life and in the lives of those surrounding her. Although *coraggio* was the critical element needed to act, it also was the foundation of faith, love, hope and determination that brought her through from difficulty to good.

Contemplating how Nonna met all types of adversity head on with *coraggio,* I realized the vital chain of events that could be evoked from the power of courage. The power imbued in courage could confer the will to live, and the will to live would spur hope of healing. Courage and hope could elicit determination to fight for healing.

Hope! Hope of healing the pain suffered in your physical body. Hope of healing the pain of the devastating losses oppressing your heart. Believe that if you can harness that hope all the strength needed for those healings will follow. I believed within the core of my being that all the benefits born of courage could help me survive this chapter of my life … to walk again … to chew and swallow food again … to live … and to live a meaningful life with the healing to love again.

Coraggio!

I wanted to shout it aloud but it was four a.m. and I was surrounded by chambers of sleeping nursing home patients. I had not yet fallen asleep because the internal mind tormentors had been especially active this dark night. But I had captured a glimmer of light sent to illuminate my soul with understanding, and with that understanding, the *courage to hope.* Now the kindling of hope had sparked an enthusiasm. With heels and elbows against the chafing rough sheets of the hospital bed, I shimmied my body as high up in the bed as I was capable. Inserting my hand through the bars of the bedrail I was able to reach a blank-paged book from the nightstand, given to me as a gift.

Thank God I was able to reach this journal. And thank God there is a pen clasped to the inside pages so it did not fall out.

I had often time been frustrated because when an urge to write came, I could not reach either paper or a pen. Or if I could reach one item of the writing duo the other would fall to the floor and I was left waiting until someone entered the room to fetch it. *It is good sign that you have both necessities for writing.* I used the electronic button on the side of the hospital bed to elevate the head section until I was almost sitting upright. I started writing and wrote, and wrote. Courage had removed my fear of bringing into consciousness the horrific details of what had occurred to my mother and Nagymama before, during and after the scene of the car accident. I wrote down every morbid, sad, grotesque, disappointing, angry, hurtful thought and feeling about the accident and the surrounding circumstances.

Wham! With both hands I slammed the covers of the book tightly shut. Courage gave me the strength to feel the pain of loss, the ache of regret for past hurtful words uttered, and for the love-acknowledging words that should have been said.

Ah-ha! All you mind-tormentors! You are ousted from my subconscious thought and onto the written page! You are trapped within the pages now. No longer are you in my mind!

Tormentors of fear, anxiety, guilt and whatever else left in the bastion of negative thought, defeated for at least the time being by the courage to fight and conquer the dreaded monsters. The dawn's light not having yet broken, I fell into an exhausted but restful sleep.

The next day was a non-apheresis dialysis day. On this first day of renewed hope the most remarkable event occurred. In later years I came to believe this event was an actual manifestation of the positive self-affirmation derived from my renewed hope.

I was lying in my nursing home bed, which was what I did on non-apheresis days. It was late afternoon and a confident young surgeon walked into my room, having finished a surgery at the nearby hospital. He paused at the end of my bed and faced me. I tugged the bed sheet up toward my neck in a subconscious effort to hide the immodesty of the thin, ill-fitting hospital gown and lack of other proper coifing. I was not expecting any medical professional or anyone else for that matter, so I nodded the suave surgeon toward my roommate. He remained at the end of my bed, examining me more from the perspective of sizing me up than from the perspective of a medical examination.

"I am here to see you. I am Dr. B. Your rheumatologist asked me to do her a favor because I owe her a favor. So I told her I would, and that is why I am here."

What does a debtor's score between my U.C.L.A. rheumatologist and this North Hollywood surgeon have to do with me?

"She asked me to perform a knee replacement surgery for you. When she told me you only had Medi-Cal insurance I declined and told her I do not perform surgery for anyone with government sponsored insurance. It is too much of a hassle to deal with the government programs. That's when she pulled out a 'favor' chit from her sleeve. She must really like you. Anyway, I did not make her any promises but I told her I would at least stop by this facility after surgery to determine whether you would even be a candidate for knee replacement surgery."

I was embarrassed by the comment the doctor made about me using public assistance.

Doesn't he know that no relative in my genealogical chart has ever used public assistance? I come from hard-working, proud stock. Doesn't he know I am unable to walk or use my arms and legs because I am debilitated by this weird neurological disease, not knowing if I can pull out of the seemingly downward spiraling drag of myasthenia gravis, and topping all, both my caretakers were recently killed ... and only under these drastic circumstances had I been signed up for public assistance? I am not a malingerer! Never in my wildest imagination would I have dreamed I would use Medi-Cal health insurance.

The surgeon rebuffed my rheumatologist's request to consider me for knee replacement surgery, telling her that he did not accept Medi-Cal patients. She asked him if he would do the favor of at least going over and talking with me. They reached an agreement on that aspect alone. I had no idea. The last thing I was thinking about was knee replacement surgery. But as promised, here he was the first afternoon of my renewed hope day. He had not rushed in on a blazing bolt of lightening as an enthusiastic angel of mercy. Adorned in work-crumbled hospital scrubs he appeared somewhat put off, begrudging being coerced into an agreement with my rheumatologist. Armed with new found courage just hours before, I embraced the concept of two total knee replacements and the prospect of walking once again.

The surgeon softened and then compassionately explained the knee replacement process, the risks, and the benefits. It was a complicated decision for me. My mother and I had worked relentlessly to heal my body and regenerate the tissues involved with my knees so that I could walk again. But with courage I could part with my mother's and my unwavering goal of walking without having to cut out and discard forever my mere twenty-something body parts. With courage I could do this by myself; without the supportive mom, a spouse, or family on this side of the continent.

By the time the surgeon left we had a plan. He agreed to accept me as a Medi-Cal patient and I agreed to get strong enough to withstand the surgery and recovery.

Employing courage realized from the prior night, the wellspring of determination, hope and healing overflowed, and miracles started to occur. Within three months my right knee was replaced. By Christmas the left knee was replaced. Marvels were unceasing! One year to the date of my mother's accidental death I stood in the hospital hall and took my first steps in three years! Was the timing coincidental? I don't think so. Did her freed and enlightened soul or being play a part in bringing about this incredible miracle as well as orchestrate the timing to assure me of her role? I had had unexpected complications following the second knee replacement surgery and was not supposed to be starting physical therapy or to be hospitalized on that anniversary date, but here I was, miracles in hand.

The scene was a conglomerate of emotions that led to sheer rapture. I sat in my wheelchair, mid-hallway of the long orthopedic surgery floor. I leaned slightly forward while the physical therapist tightened the wide, thickly-woven safety belt around my waist. I wore two hospital gowns, one tied in the front and the second worn in reverse for modesty's sake. Nonetheless the standard-sized belt was too long for my thin waist and it was yanked until my protruding hip bones were visible from under the gowns. The physical therapist forced hand levers to safely lock in place my wheelchair.

"I'm ready. I … I want to try by myself." I stared straight ahead from my seated position, plastic-soled, quilted bootie slippers planted flatly at equal distance on the floor, with the focused attention of an Olympic skier readying herself for a perfect-form burst out of the starting gate.

The physical therapist, who had sounded cautiously worried minutes before, had changed to a tone of cautiously optimistic at my determined tenor. "Okay, if you think you can do it, I have you gripped tightly by the belt. If you feel as if you are going to buckle let me know and I will lower you slowly back into the chair, holding you by the belt. I won't let you fall."

I tightened the quadriceps muscles around my knees and thighs as previously instructed by the physical therapist and started to push myself up out of the seat of the wheelchair. I reached out to the platform walker perched resolutely in front of me. I pushed with my thighs and pulled with my arms. I was part way elevated, meaning in plain, crude terms, my bottom had lifted off! I felt sharp pains and the grating of crepitus cartilage against jagged bones within the joints. Simultaneous was the sick sound of cracking in my fingers, wrists and elbows as the decrepit joints and feeble muscles tried to work at pulling and bearing the weight of my upper body. I grabbed the handles of the walker and pulled my rear into a more erect position. I was upright! *ARRRRGH!* The pain in the surgery sore new knees and upper body joints was incredible; but I was standing upright all on my own! My thigh muscles started twitching, already wobbling with fatigue. *C'mon. You can do this. C'mon legs, you can do this!* **Do it for Mom. Do it for Nagymama!** I shifted my weight as if to brush off the quivering.

"Great, Lisa. Now try to lift your chin so you are looking forward. There … that's it. Now tuck your butt in some more. Keep looking forward." The physical therapist sounded immeasurably impressed that the two of us had accomplished the amazing feat of standing at the first try in three years. The excitement in her voice further motivated me.

I pulled my head up until my chin was tucked and parallel to the floor. I heaved my shoulders back to further improve my posture. I looked ahead at the features of the distant hallway. Moving only my eyes so as not to throw off my balance I glanced from side to side at the hospital corridor surroundings. After sitting at wheelchair level for three years, the viewpoint from five feet height was perceptively odd. It was mind-blowing how differently surroundings looked from a standing position. My mind had automatically changed its perspective during those seated years and I felt as if I was engaged in one of those sensory deception chamber experiments or the Hall of Mirrors from a fifty-cents childhood county carnival show.

"How're ya doin? Do you need to sit down?" The physical therapist asked almost disingenuously, as if not wanting to concede the phenomenal achievement at this level.

No, no, no! I am never going to sit down again!

The physical therapist did not wait for me to answer in the affirmative, and instead launched into, "When you are ready I want you to shift all your weight to the right leg then lift the left leg and move your left foot forward."

I focused my mind entirely on shifting my body's weight to my right leg. With forced concentration I urged my brain to signal the left foot. *Lift … c'mon l-i-f-t.* I felt my left foot lift slightly off the ground. The pain in the tissues surrounding my three-month-old right knee screamed in protest as all of my hundred pound body mass was foisted onto it. Every joint in my upper body cracked and groaned as I tried to bear some of the body weight with my upper torso. My right shoulder snapped slightly out of place in its joint space and I heard the dislocating "pop" ricochet through my carcass into my eardrum. The left leg muscles shook furiously under its valiant effort. Sweat copiously sprang in all its usual places. I forced the half-lifted, half-sliding, slippered foot about one and a half inches forward before it gave way to gravity's great beckon. My first step!

Emotion-fed adrenalin surged through my body and dashed away any cognizance of pain or muscle fatigue. I forced my mind to repeat the procedure, this time with opposite leg and foot. The step forward was greater—<u>two</u> inches on this second attempt!

My body shook but this time with the gushing wellspring of joyous sobbing. *I can't believe I walked two steps!* I was bent forward in hunched formation and tears splattered on the hallway tiles beneath me. The physical therapist realized the tears and waves of trembling were from sobs and she too began to shed tears.

A puddle of tears collected on that hallway floor under my platform walker. Tears of joy from me...*upright <u>me</u>* actually standing on my own two feet! And tears from the physical therapist gripping the safety belt strapped to my waist and from nurses who flocked from the nursing station and patient rooms to witness my miracle! I am absolutely positive there were tears from heaven in that puddle, too. My mother had striven with every bit of her earthly being so that I might walk again. Here on the first anniversary of her death, I could deliver to her and to Nagymama a more meaningful gift than any to wherever their beautiful souls alighted! Did that gift of "Lisa's little steps" make up for the less than optimal last moments we spent together and not knowing the moments should be coveted as the last? Absolutely! *Look at me, Mom! Look at me, Nagymama! It is everything we worked toward! I know you are both looking down at me!*

As I looked up from the growing puddle to the painted ceiling of the corridor I sent the mental message to Mom and Nagymama with the exuberance of a kid on her first bike ride without training wheels. I delivered the mental message with a heart swell of gratitude and pride. All concern about them not knowing the depth of my love and appreciation dissolved with the intensity of love I silently expressed at this moment. *I know you both continue to work your miracles for me from heaven! Thank you! You are amazing!*

What did it matter that I had to spend Christmas in the hospital? I had been given the greatest Christmas present: two working knees and the ability to walk again! The Christmas Carol I sang aloud was my own version of Alvin and the Chipmunks, "All I Want for Christmas is My Two Front Teeth." I switched several of the lyrics to fit my occasion and burst aloud with mischievous smile, "All I want for Christmas are my two new knees ... *ta da*... my two new knees ... *ta da* ... yes, my two new knees!"

And *I had* received those two new knees by Christmas. What did it matter that I had taken public transportation all by myself the morning of surgery and remained alone during the hospitalization, my immediate family thousands of miles away? It didn't matter. It was less than one year from that desolate nursing home night when *coraggio*, heard as a whisper, rebounded with a fury that produced miracles. And one of the miracles spinning off from the resurgence of *coraggio* was that I could walk!

"*Coraggio, Leeza. Coraggio.*"

How important were those words Nonna spoke. This simple woman, formally educated only through the seventh grade because she had to leave school to earn money to help support her family. This modest woman, meagerly existing on a blue-collar, shop worker widow's pension. What could this simple, modest woman possibly offer to the granddaughter she loved so dearly? She could offer her life-lessons in courage learned by living through her own difficult challenges, joyous celebrations, and agonizing situations. *Coraggio's* faith and hope helped her survive. *Coraggio* produced fortitude and forged determination. *Coraggio* fostered a positive outlook and illuminated the path toward purpose-filled direction.

"*Coraggio, Leeza. Coraggio.*"

How often in my life I would envision her saying those words to me, deep set eyes fixed straight ahead in her soft but willful tone. Determination, strength, hope, will to live and healing cascaded from courage. Her example taught me more than a paramount life lesson; it was a life-*saving* lesson. Her encouragement bore stubbornness in me to take charge of the aspects of my life I could control. *Coraggio* saved my life.

My dire predicament that frightful nursing home night forced me on my knees, bowing before the face of God. I realized it may have taken brutal dramatic circumstances to force a total surrender of my *testadura* will to that of God's will. That total desperation, exhaustion and fear that lonely dark night, virtually laid prone, forehead pressed against a cold, stone floor with no other human available to rescue me was necessary to reach within my being. The earnest internal search reaped discovery of who I truly was and why I had to live through that particular moment in those particular circumstances.

Part of that discovery was the inexhaustible strength I possessed with which I could achieve almost any goal. For the first time the window wiped clean to view with clarity my true life purpose. I strapped on courage to yank free from the vortex of despair and armed with the elucidative discoveries moved in forward motion to fulfill my undeniable life purpose.

Coraggio enables me to walk on my two feet today. *Coraggio* is the reason for remarkable and successful careers as an attorney, advocate, super-aunt, policy advisor to the Michigan Senate, policy staffer to Governor John Engler, and currently as a state administrative law judge. *Coraggio* enables me to wake up each morning with a "gratitude attitude", with "seize the day" determination and smile perpetuation throughout the day.

I do not say this whimsically or without personal employ. Without *coraggio* this book may never have manifested. Lying within me for years was the inner-realization of how my experiences with physical pain and emotional grief were connected to the importance of appreciating each present moment. Inner stirrings, moments of inspiration and occasional strong urgings consistently poked at my conscience and soul. But I was distracted by other versions of "saving the world" or by the self-doubt whisperings of "who cares about your stories?" or "God gave you many talents but did not give you the talent for writing." It is with prayers and *coraggio* that I fought against the negative self-talk and life distractions, to stubbornly plod along for twenty years until the writings began to flow and appear on my computer screen.

It is interesting when I look back on my life situations where, if viewed by the external world, may have elicited a grimace or pity. But for me, those occasions of intense pain and debility provided opportunity for marvelously rich internal shifts, and opportunity to sit still and actually write parts of this book.

I had four back-to-back major ankle surgeries mandating more than nine months of absolutely no weight bearing or walking. Sounds unbearable, eh? However, when I look back, it was the writing done at that time, half-propped, half lying in bed with laptop on tray table over my torso and leg elevated, that afforded the inertia needed to finally move this book toward reality.

Thus it is with earnest purpose that I press upon you the Old World life lessons taught to me by a simple, modest, sweet Italian grandmother. Her stories overlaid upon my stories, unfolded to en*courage* you and spark the passions of determination, hope, faith, love, purpose and healing.

For whatever challenge or heartbreak you may be weightily enduring, do not become dis*couraged*; do not give up! The frigid, dark night of the soul, frighteningly devoid of light may be needed to discover who you truly are to discover your undeniable life purpose. And if not the "a-ha!" of the grand scheme, pain may pull you to a sudden screeching halt or debilitation may force you into a stillness needed to reflect on that very instant in time so that you can experience that single moment, not wishing you had your old body back, not worrying about whether the pain will ever go away, and perhaps reach an understanding of the reason you are in that moment and truly appreciate that moment whether externally the circumstances could be viewed as negative.

Courage is always there to afford the bravery needed to take an honest assessment of our inner-self, the forthright internal review necessary for self-discovery; and courage is always there to carry self-discovery forward to indomitably fulfill your life purpose. Have courage to hang in there long enough for realization to manifest. Do not cut short the process, as painful or hopeless as it may seem, lest realization be thwarted.

Have courage to keep your mind and heart open, as frustrating as it may be to guard your mind and heart against negative thoughts or anger, lest purpose be dashed. I am as tough and stubborn as they come. Perhaps it took that horrific dark night of the soul to force me prone before the throne of God and beg for His help and grace to see what purpose there was to my being in the terrifically unjust and agonizingly painful moment; His wisdom to discern what purpose the experience could have for helping me and others in the future; His strength to accept my undeniable purpose and work indomitably toward its fulfillment.

Whether you believe in God, the Universe's plan, a Greater Power or Source with whom you may recognize and connect or none of the aforementioned, all you need to survive chronic, serious illness or devastating loss lies within.

Courage serves as the survival tools' foundation.

Courage is:

- Maintaining hope even when the future appears dim.
- Moving forward even when you feel despair or overwhelmed.
- Discovering a sense of purpose from a tangled web of life circumstances.
- Finding peace when the end of life is staring you in the face.
- Helping another find peace when the end of their life is staring you in the face.

Chapter 10
Willow Branches

Willow branch baskets were the handicraft of my Great-Grandfather Genaro's artistic hands. The baskets appeared in several of Nonna's stories playing both minor and major cameos. Nonna told the story of how her father often walked his handiwork to surrounding village markets, the proceeds from their sale provided for him and his young family in Pedivigliano, Italy.

A frequently repeated story was how Nonna's mother carried on her head one of her husband's baskets filled with figs to sell. The figs were magnificent as only the Mediterranean variety can boast, bulging globes of royal purple hue topped lightly with a splash of chartreuse, the fruit would fetch a handsome and much-needed income.

The distance to the neighboring town markets was great and the road uneasy. Needing to cross a river to continue the path, Nonna's mother turned her bare foot on an unseen stone on the river's bed and stumbled, causing the basket on top her head unsettled and figs to tumble into the shallow water and mud of the river's edge. Fearing her income lost as the fruit was displeasingly dented, misshapen and dirty, Nonna's mother sat at the river's sloped edge and began to quietly weep.

Nearby laborers witnessed the mishap and felt sorry for the young woman. They reassured her that the figs were fine; rinsing them in the river and dangling the purple globes by their stems, the blazing sun as background, to aid her inspection. They offered to buy every fig, animatedly exclaiming it would be the best lunch they had eaten in weeks.

Nonna's mother went home with an empty basket. The cloth she had used to line the basket no longer cuddled valuable fruit, but instead clutched a handful of precious coins. The seeming disaster not only produced earnings for her family, she had been spared the long journey and hours spent at market, and returned early to finish her many home chores.

Nonna's tone emanated affectionate pride as she explained how during the early summer her father scouted, selectively gathered and stored flexible willow branches. Thicker, strong braches would serve as the supporting foundation, and thinner, nimble branches would be woven inside and outside of the foundational skeleton to construct the utilitarian masterpieces.

During the winter months of diminishing daylight hours and decreased crop maintenance, her father carefully soaked the select foundational willow branches, along with more slender, threader branches. Nonna expressed how vividly she recalled those winter nights, watching her father as he sat close to the fire in their tiny, rustic home, his quick, nimble fingers weaving the wet threader twigs efficiently around the foundational branches to create various sized and shaped baskets.

Lezione Uno: Coraggio, Leeza (Lesson One: Courage, Lisa)

Typically three malleable branches were twisted into six prongs, the spokes of which were bent into a basket shape and dried to form. The six strong, stiff branches served as the form around which were laced slender, twig-like branches to fill in the basket's shape. Some of the creations were large, sturdy oval baskets to carry laundry to the river for washing. Others were medium-sized, tall-sided baskets with flat bottoms to place upon the head and carry figs to market. There were also smaller shallow baskets to fetch and store eggs.

The willow basket of my great-grandfather's adored hands perfectly symbolizes the seven lessons Nonna imparted to me about living life despite formidable challenges with chronic illness, pain, and loss. In this analogy, *Coraggio* is *Lezione Uno* (Lesson One), akin to the slender, malleable willow branch. The branch may appear insignificant and less potent in its suppleness. Yet, as this branch is woven in between each of the six skeletal posts, it binds them together as a whole and gives strength and support to the basket's end shape and purpose. In the summers of our lives we gather and store the supportive instrument so that in the winters of our life we can use it as bedrock with which to give shape and provide platform for our life purpose.

Interlocked among the slender threaded branches are the six foundational branches. In the analogy these six branches are six aspects that stem from courage and are vital to living life with *gusto* (vivaciously) despite adversity. Herein lies Nonna's remaining six life lessons:

Lezione Due (Lesson Two)—the courage to attain and maintain a positive and take charge attitude

Lezione Tre (Lesson Three)—the courage to love yourself, to receive, love and to love others after loss or hurt

Lezione Quattro (Lesson Four)—the courage to believe in faith, hope, prayers, healing and miracles

Lezione Cinque (Lesson Five)—the courage to discover new perspectives and approaches to dealing with physical and emotional pain

Lezione Sei & Lezione Sette (Lesson Six & Lesson Seven)—the courage to grieve the loss of a beloved and the courage to honor the end of life.

The six foundational willow branches may become slightly misplaced or split by bumps or burdensome load, but the binding branches of courage will never allow the basket to break. So will courage securely support you through life's bumps or burdens.

More than a precious artistic masterpiece, the willow basket serves another purpose, which is a repository of life's belongings and treasures. How will you form the shape and strength of your willow basket? What purpose will your willow basket serve? With what items and what quantity will you fill your willow basket?

Call on *coraggio* for the determination to take charge of your life and the strength to shape your life to its fulfilling purpose.

Courage is:
- The foundation of living with *gusto* despite chronic illness, pain and loss.

Lezione Due: Il Malocchio
(Lesson Two: The Evil Eye)

The Courage to Take Charge of the Aspects of Life You Can Control

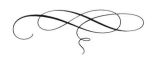

CHAPTER 11

The Evil Eye

THROUGHOUT MY LIFE NONNA TOLD ME STORIES ABOUT SUPERSTITIOUS ITALIAN folk who inflicted vengeful curses. *Superstiziosi* (superstition) was believed along with and as solemnly as any religious doctrine in Nonna's southern Calabria region of Italy. Accordingly, Nonna told *Il Malocchio!* (The Evil Eye) stories with a serious tone and credulous face. In her tales the characters exacting evil were not *streganonni* (witches), rather they were spiteful or jealous townsfolk seeking revenge or conveying their displeasure.

As a little girl I sat with wide-eyed captivity for Nonna's tales of the cursed.

"It happened that an elderly mother thought *her* son should marry the town's most popular girl. This mother was outraged;

instead of marrying *her* son, the girl had agreed to marry the first guy who proposed to her!" Nonna made the pronouncement in exaggerated urgent tone to signal commencement of a catastrophic legend.

Nonna's eyes were fierce with imagined vengeance, her voice reaching a punitive pitch. "*Ohhhhh* … this old lady was *aaaaaan-gry*. She was fit to be tied! So she set out to 'fix' the guy who had proposed in advance of her son's proposal."

My young-girl mind conjured a four-foot, stooped widow, squeezed in a heavy black cotton dress, despite the hot Calabrese sun, setting out on her vendetta pilgrimage. I recognized this particular oft told, Evil Eye story. *It was going to be bad for the impetuous fool-in-love guy* … The prickling at the back of my neck signaled growing eeriness.

Nonna interrupted her jaw-clenched serious tone for a moment to interject her personal opinion with an air of righteous authority. "After all, everyone in the town knew *her* son had his eye on the girl first."

As Nonna returned to her scary story-telling composure, my young imagination became fully engaged. In my mind I could see the old, vengeful Italian woman in black cotton, stocking-covered legs appearing from under the concealing folds of her heavy black skirt as she shuffled gradually along uneven stones that paved the narrow street. I heard the scuffle of tattered, bulky black leather shoes. Street dust, unsettled from the worn leather soles that had scraped against the arid stone road, filled in the cracks of the worn leather and filled the gap between the bulging, laced ties. The taupe powder gathered on the rolls of the heavy black cotton stockings as they bunched at her bloated ankles. She pauses. The old woman's neck apparently fused to her stiffened hunched back, twists only slightly. With the stiff rotation of the head I see the braided bun of grey hair follow the movement. Her face turns toward the door of the unsuspecting victim. Suspense thickens. But it is the sight of her eyes that cause me to shudder—cold, deep, black that connotes evil. It was the penetrating black eyes that moved slowly toward the victim's house scanning for its prey. Once locked in to the malevolent-eyed sights there is no escape! The frightful black eyes cast an evil spell; further propelled by an undecipherable full-lipped utterance and right-hand gesticulation. The impetuous, fool-in-love guy is screwed.

I was terrified! I knew the narration was merely one of the "Old Country" tales, but the combination of Nonna's fierce storytelling and my lively imagination produced the feeling of some creepy-crawly, million-legged, hairy thing crawling up the back of my neck and into my ear to hatch its young-lings. *It's okay; it happened long ago; rid the creeps with a full-body shake-off.*

According to Nonna the curse-caster could place a curse that was short-lived but devastating. Or the curse-caster could place a curse to plague you for the rest of your life and continue on through your progeny. As I grew older, my curiosity was able to overcome the terrified mesmerism. Of course, I just wanted to know the good stuff.

"Nonna, really, just how contorted were his legs and arms after the Evil Eye got him? Was his body all contorted for the rest of his life?"

And with further maturity I was more intrigued to learn why a person was cursed than what gruesome tragedy happened to the cursed. I interrupted Nonna mid-story and asked, "Nonna, what could that guy possibly have done? I mean, what could he have done so horrendous to provoke such devastating ill wishes?"

As an adult, I seriously doubted the authenticity of *il malocchio* power. I admit my childhood-instilled terror induced a slight prickling around the black Italian forearm hairs. But I reasoned that in actuality the cause had a scientific explanation or coincidence, not an evil-doing spell.

As she was in her late 80s and had lived far from the superstition-abiding land of Italy for seventy years, I had no idea

Nonna continued a fervent belief in curses, much less herself a caster of *il malocchio*.

I called Nonna one day and she answered in a panicky gasp. "Oh Leeza!"

O dear Lord; some relative has gone to heaven. I feared the worst from the breathless sound of her voice.

"I killed him. *O Madon'*, I killed him!" she cried.

It took me a minute to figure out what was going on because she was speaking rapidly, partly in Italian and partly in English, interjecting "*O Madon!*" with despairing moans throughout the mixed language sentences. Part of the delay in my comprehension of the situation was because the idea of my sweet Nonna actually killing any human was incomprehensible.

"*Il malocchio!*" she stammered at me impatiently as I was trying to pull the English translation from the right side of my brain. "The *curse, Leeza!*" she stammered emphatically, exasperated because I had not instantly understood.

I could see in my mind Nonna's posture at that exact moment. She was sitting forward, her face was tight with fret and the hand that was not holding the phone to her ear was firmly grasping the padded arm of her velour lounge chair. Everyone in the family recognized Nonna's panic pose.

"*Aspetto, Nonna,*" ("Wait, Nonna.") I begged, thinking it best to halt her by addressing her in her native language.

Eventually I got her to slow down her speech enough to tell me the story, mostly in English although she continued to groan with guilt and invoke the name of the Blessed Virgin Mary after every few sentences.

As told, the man who lived directly behind Nonna placed fill-dirt in the low-lying areas of his backyard, spreading the recess-filling dirt flush against the fence they shared. It sounded like a good idea for residents of the small blue-collar backyards subject to Lake St. Clair's high water table flooding. The problem with the neighbor's project was that the level of dirt he accomplished was higher than the ground level on Nonna's side of the fence. As a consequence, at the next heavy rain, water ran downward from the higher level of his yard and flooded the back of Nonna's yard. Perhaps the resulting mini-lake that was once Nonna's backyard could have been anticipated by a neighbor building up the ground level of his backyard. Regardless of the neighbor's intentions, Nonna was so upset with the man she placed a monstrous curse on him and his backyard.

The next evening the shrill siren and bright lights of an ambulance caught her attention. Through the backyard fence she saw the ambulance stop at his house. The neighbor's garage and the back of the his house obscured most of her view of what was taking place at the neighbor's front door and parked ambulance. Nonna asked a neighbor lady friend to call a second lady friend who lived on the same street as the man to find out what happened. The lady friend reported back to Nonna that the man had been taken from his house by ambulance and had died! Nonna resolutely, and with full-blown guilt and remorse believed it was her backyard curse that had killed him.

"Leeza, I did not mean for *il malocchio* to kill him. I just wanted to give his backyard some little *afflitto* (affliction) for what he did to me; honest, Leeza." Her confession was weighted with overwhelming guilt.

I wanted to soothe Nonna's guilt by convincing her there was no power in *il malocchio*. The problem with debunking *il malocchio* was I did not want to eviscerate an evidently important tool she used to take charge of her life. I would be telling an elderly lady of limited physical and financial capabilities that the means she used to feel she had control over aspects of her life was non-effectual. It was a difficult dilemma to resolve.

The tale appears to be about a negative action taken and negative result achieved. But there is a positive moral to be derived.

Nonna had reached far back to her Old County practices and illustrated an important lesson: "Take charge of what you can control and let go of the rest."

As Nonna told the full story, she explained that heavy rains had pooled in a lower than ground level basin area between her backyard and the backyard of the neighbor behind her lot. A pond formed in both of their backyards, the back chain fence dividing the pool almost evenly. Nonna clarified that her initial plan was to build fill-dirt to the same level raised by the backyard neighbor. With both backyards at the same level, her backyard would not flood.

As Nonna had moved forward with her initial plan she realized that at 80-plus years old she could not shovel the one ton of topsoil needed to raise the level sufficiently. She had not wanted to bother her grandsons to shovel and haul dirt for hours nor could she afford to have someone place the dirt. So she had decided to take charge in a manner in which she *was* able. She had taken the long-handled hoe that served to steady her thin five-foot frame as she traversed the uneven brick and sod of her garden path. She had stood there in her backyard facing the back of the neighbor's house, her hand around the hoe's handle that rose above her head. With a determination akin to Moses, tall wooden staff in hand, preparing to part the Red Sea, Nonna spoke the words of the curse and sealed it with the hand gestures. With one final flick of the back of her hand, upward over her throat, under her chin and outward until her arm was extended, she flung *il malocchio* toward her enemy. And with the flinging of that curse Nonna had taken charge of her situation.

You may believe that you have no control over chronic illness in your life. You may feel that day after day you feel pain, your body deteriorates, and there is nothing you can do about it. When I think back to *il malocchio* I fervently disagree. I believe each person has within them the resources necessary to take charge of at least some part of their health, even if struggling with chronic illness. My frail 86-year-old Italian grandmother found a way, even if it may have been extreme, to believe she had taken charge of her flooded backyard situation. I do not mean to advocate for going out and flinging curses.

The point is there is always some aspect of a situation over which you have control. Ban the doubting thoughts, the anxious feelings, and all the internal and external distractions. Become still for a moment. Look beyond the illness and there you will discover manageable features of your health and your life. In that moment of stillness and discovery become aware of what stirs within you. Identify the resources that lay within, the resources you can take hold to manage those features of health and life. With both arms outstretched in beckoning gesture, call forth the resources and sound the call until it reverberates in every tissue within you. Apply the gathered resources full-heartedly as bravely and readily as possible, all the while letting the passersby and heavens hear the cry: *Coraggio!*

With courage it is possible to:

- Recognize there are elements of your illness and components of your health over which you have control.
- Acknowledge you have inner and external resources with which you can take charge of your health.
- Acknowledge you have inner and external resources with which you can take charge of your life.
- Apply your resources to take charge of your health.
- Apply your resources to take charge of your life.

CHAPTER 12

Grab Courage, Take Charge!

Uɴɪᴛᴇᴅ Sᴛᴀᴛᴇs Sᴇɴᴀᴛᴏʀ Jᴏʜɴ McCᴀɪɴ, ɪɴ ʜɪs ʙᴏᴏᴋ *Wʜʏ Cᴏᴜʀᴀɢᴇ Matters: The Way to a Braver Life,* tells the story about a young Green Beret soldier named Roy Benevidez. As Senator McCain tells the story, Master Sergeant Benevidez volunteered to evacuate twelve men who were encircled by Vietnamese troops and under a barrage of gunfire. When the evacuation helicopter reached the men, four were dead and all remaining eight were wounded badly enough to be immobile. With ferocious courage Benevidez jumped out of the helicopter and ran toward the wounded. Before he reached them he was shot in the face, the arm and the head. Incredibly, he continued getting up and running until he made it to the men. He applied medical treatment and even more incredibly got all but one aboard the evacuation helicopter. He reached the last man, the team leader, the man with classified documents. The helicopter pilot was fatally shot and as a result the helicopter crashed upside down and started to burn. Even though Master Sergeant Benevidez was seriously wounded, he managed to get the wounded men out of the burning helicopter. But the enemy kept closing in. With ingenuity and superhuman strength and bravery Benevidez tended to and encouraged the wounded, summoned air and ship strikes, and held off the enemy, including engaging one Vietcong in hand to hand fight to the death, for six hours until another evacuation attempt was successful. All in all, Sergeant Benevidez suffered seven gunshot wounds (serious enough to spill his intestines) twenty-eight shrapnel wounds, and bayonet stabs to his arms.

How do you explain courage? Why do some people possess courage while others give up or fall prey to a hopeless dismay? McCain reminds us that Winston Churchill stated:

"Courage is the first of human qualities because it guarantees all the others."

McCain states: "We are taught to understand, correctly, that courage is not the absence of fear, but the capacity for action despite our fears."

McCain posits that courage is a combination virtue, an active conscience, a love of dignity, a sense of duty that provokes the experience of shame when it is disobeyed, a perspective that ranks the objects of courage higher than its penalties, a capacity for outrage, a seeking nature, hope, and the desire and willingness to have courage, but always fear. In other words, you must be afraid of someone or something in order for courage to exist.

So, do we have to sustain the horrors of Sergeant Master Benevidez in order to display courage? How much physical suffering,
emotional grieving do we need endure to be a hero?

McCain writes:

Suffering is not, by itself, courage; fearing what we
choose to suffer is.

At twenty-five years old I could have looked at my life
and only seen the losses: I could no longer walk and for years
had to use a wheelchair full-time; I could no longer partici-
pate in my two favorite sports: running and skiing; I was not
in medical school despite many years of study and striving;
I was not, as were many friends my age, falling in love, getting married, having children, and buying the white-picket-
fenced home; and the two women with whom I had lived,
had shared my daily thoughts, had loved the most and relied
on as caregivers had suddenly died, leaving a huge, aching
void in my physical, emotional and spiritual life. Or, I could
look at my life and focus on the good and abundance in my
life. I had two legs; the nerves in my two legs had a working connection with the brain and were not paralyzed; there
were sports other than running and downhill skiing, swimming for one, I could try; my brain continued in its high
functioning state, and with such blessed mental capacity I
could study and attain a profession from which I could support myself, even while waiting to become strong enough
to be in medical school; I had angelic and generous friends;
and I had the opportunity to foster the legacy of my two
grandmothers: pride in heritage and importance of family,
and to foster the legacy of my mother: joyful living.

I had a choice. I could choose each morning to dress myself in the list of negatives and wear those negatives throughout

my day, see myself and greet each opportunity and encounter with a self-pitying and debilitating attitude of "I can't and I don't have"; or I could choose each morning to dress myself in the list of positives and wear those positives throughout my day, see myself and greet each opportunity and encounter with a self-affirming and forward moving attitude of "I can and I am grateful for all I have."

In the wheelchair-dependent days after my mother and grandmother died I chose to focus on the positives in my life and to pursue a next-step-forward-moving action with passion. The first thing on the list was bilateral knee replacement surgery with the belief I would walk again.

While the replacement of knees process took place I enrolled in a Child, Family and Marriage Counseling Masters Degree program at California State University, Northridge wherein I could arrange wheelchair van transportation to the classroom building from my apartment. The plan was to pursue a professional counseling license while in a wheelchair with the goal of attaining a profession I could perform from a wheelchair if necessary. Part of the forward moving plan was to tell myself each day, *See beauty in all that surrounds you. Be joyous toward others in every situation. Mom lived her life in that manner; you witnessed the deep joy she felt within and you saw the overwhelming, uplifting affect her joyous encounter had on others.*

Nonna taught me the lesson of having the courage to take charge of the aspects of life you could control. But how does a person take that general concept and apply it to the unique aspects of one's own life? The national Arthritis Foundation has developed a self-help brochure entitled, "Take Control of your Arthritis, Take Charge of your Life." Local chapters of the Arthritis Foundation have volunteer speakers who talk about the concept of taking charge of your life through self-help. I wholeheartedly agree with their concept and offer my own version of controlling your health by taking charge of any of the aspects you can. Grab courage! Take charge! The battle cry: *Coraggio*!

With courage you can:

- Recognize the fear that may be holding you back from taking charge of your health or a life situation.
- Move forward despite fear.

CHAPTER 13

Take Charge of the Aspects of Health Care Within Your Control

You MAY NOT BE ABLE TO CHANGE THE FACT THAT YOU HAVE A TERMINAL diagnosis or may not be able to control the chronic nature of your illness, but you *can* control many aspects of your health care. One way to take charge is to recognize you have health care choices—a variety of healing treatments or additional health practitioner opinions. The following story, oft told by Nonna in the half century since its occurrence, illustrates how even though a medical situation may appear hopeless, there is always an opportunity for a different approach if you believe and search for it.

Nonna raised my father Pasquale in a sturdy two-flat structure typical of the east side Detroit neighborhood. In the late 1930s this neighborhood of European immigrants was mostly residential, interspersed with small shops and churches. St. Philip's Catholic Church and attached school was one of those churches and where Pasquale walked to elementary school and daily Mass.

The vicinity also contained a metal-stamping factory and railroad tracks whose inherently intriguing yet dangerous qualities beckoned adventuresome, curious boys. One of many automotive parts foundries indigenous to Detroit, the Budd Company's metal stamping plant, smelted ore to produce metals that were then stamped into automotive doors, side panels and bumpers. Not only did the plant provide a livelihood for more than a hundred members of the community, the architecture of its building was built in the 1920s to resemble Philadelphia's Independence Hall. The smokestacks behind the majestic clock tower churned billows of black soot as tons of metal was separated from its ore. As a courtesy to its neighbors, as hundreds of workers filed out of the building at the end of the afternoon shift, the Budd Company sounded a shrill siren alerting residents to the imminent blasts of soot-laden clouds.

Another byproduct of the smelting process was glowing red hot, fused glassy material that turned black when cooled. The smoldering slag was dumped in the open lots adjacent to the 85-acre foundry compound.

Can you imagine the wide-eyed fascination of the seven-year-old neighborhood boys as they watched the succession of dump trucks, feeling the thunderous rumbling of their heavy steel elevating beds loaded with cargo, while the enthralling trucks drove slowly in a straight line lifting the tailgate of its dump container just enough to drop a deep wake of smoldering slag. The dump trucks created a design of enticing rows; mounded, steaming, almost shimmering, black. Succulent temptation for my father Pasquale and his friends? Yes! And it was all open and available to them as soon as the dump trucks drove out of sight to the back of the monstrous building for another fill-up.

"*Presto!*" (Hurry!) "*Andiamo!* (Let's go!) Before the dump trucks return!"

To Pasquale, only about seven years old, peril was inconceivable. But the thrill of a dare was palpable. Pasquale and his friends dashed across Connor Avenue to the rows of freshly laid stinky black mounds. How could he have known he was moments away from suffering the life-threatening and losing end of a dare?

"Let's see if you can jump and make it to the other side of this big pile of ash!"

Pasquale's deep-set, brown eyes surveyed the situation. The boys were facing the rows, width-wise. There was a narrow path between each row. All he had to do was get up enough speed and height to make it over the mound to the path between it and the next mounded row. Better yet, this particular mound, laid first, no longer had steam rising off the top. Pasquale got a running start and leapt with all his might, emitting an "Ummph!" for extra height.

He hurtled his body, his skinny legs continuing their running motion in air, hoping for any extra momentum. *It looks like I am going to make it!* A victory smile started to grow on his face as he started to descend.

Suddenly, the smile dropped as fast as his body dropped. He realized the super strength he had been proudly exhibiting was going to accelerate him not only over the pile to the clear path, but further, into the next row of debris. He began flailing his arms in a backward motion as to slow the forward accelerating forces. Although succeeding in the feat of hurdling the mound, he lost in the effort to stop short of the next mound, landing several inches deep in ash of the next row. That row of slag had been more recently removed from the foundry and dumped. Under the guise of a slight top layer of blackened ash were several inches of glowing red, sizzling slag. The thick leather shoes his shoemaker grandfather had lovingly handcrafted for him miraculously protected his feet from the temperature of the slag, yet still hot enough to melt glass. But the burning ooze adhered to the unprotected skin above his shoes.

Pasquale instinctively ran into a cool puddle of water. He stood there, ankles immersed, shrieking in pain as the clinging slag sizzled through human skin to viciously devastate underlying flesh as if determined to excoriate to the bone. How he made it from the Budd Company puddle to his grandparents' bed in the lower flat remains a blur.

Typical of their European immigrant neighborhood in the early 1940s, the family physician made house calls. Italian was the primary language spoken among Pasquale's parents and grandparents in their east side Detroit home. The Italian-speaking *dottore* (*doctor*), Dr. Rizzo, rushed to their home. Shaking his head at the sight of Pasquale's badly burned ankles, he applied an ointment and wrapped several layers of cotton gauze around each ankle, while Pasquale, with all the bravery of a seven-year-old, whimpered softly. The *dottore* straightened from bending over the bed of his small patient and turned toward his mother (Nonna) and somberly instructed her to keep the ointment and wrap intact until he visited the following day. Within two days the blisters oozed thick yellow liquid, and combined with angry bloody flesh signaled the ugly threat of infection.

The *dottore* arrived as usual and began unwrapping Pasquale's bandages. Nonna and her mother Giuseppina stood against the wall of the bedroom silently surveying every move of the *dottore* as he bent over the young boy, now moaning as fever was mercifully dimming his reality. The *dottore* looked up from the horrendous sight and delivered the dreadful news to Nonna in Italian. If the damaged tissue was not improved by the time he arrived tomorrow Pasquale would have to undergo surgery to amputate his legs from mid-calf down so as to avoid a fatal infection from spreading. Unable to speak through her sobs, Nonna nodded while her mother, Giuseppina resolutely held her at her elbow. The *dottore* applied an even thicker layer of ointment, wrapped fresh gauze around the burned area and repeated his instruction to leave the ointment-soaked bandage intact.

As soon as the *dottore* walked out the door Giuseppina rushed to the bed where Pasquale lay and hurriedly unwrapped the *dottore's* bandages.

"No! *O Dio!*" Nonna shrieked and cried in horror. "*Ferma, Mama!*" (Stop, Mother!)

A loud, emotion-packed argument ensued between Nonna and her mother Giuseppina.

Nonna: "Stop unwrapping the bandages! You heard what the doctor said! We have to leave the bandages alone!"

Giuseppina: "The doctor's treatment isn't working! Pasquale's burns are only getting worse!"

Nonna: "We cannot touch the bandages! We have to do just as the doctor instructed!"

Giuseppina: "We cannot leave those bandages as they are! God, help us! Blessed Virgin, help us!"

Giuseppina left the putrefying flesh exposed to fresh air while she rushed outside behind the flat. She was a healer in her own right, applying fervent prayer and natural remedies instead of what was considered modern medicine of the time. She scoured the small patch of earth within the tiny backyard, searching for the long, deep green leaves of the plaintan plant. Not satisfied with the quantity or quality in her backyard, she crossed over into the nearby open lot, and searched, bent over through weeds and grass until she harvested an ample, robust plaintan supply. To those who did not know better, plaintan was mistaken for a dandelion or regarded as a nuisance weed, proliferating in lawns and yards. But Giuseppina knew of and believed in its healing properties. She took the fresh leaves, directly applied several to the damaged flesh, and plastered them loosely against Pasquale's ankles with a wide weave gauze. She softly uttered solemn prayers in Italian throughout the procedure.

Shortly before the *dottore* arrived the next day, Giuseppina secretively removed the plaintan and rewrapped Pasquale's ankles with the *dottore's* gauze.

What would be the *dottore's* verdict about amputation now? Would he discover Giuseppina's alternative treatment? Nonna and Giuseppina stood silently, not daring to breathe.

Then the *dottore* muttered softly in Italian, "Hmmm. The wound seems ever so slightly better. Let us wait until tomorrow to make any amputation decision."

Again, as soon as the *dottore* exited the doorstep, Giuseppina was ridding Pasquale's legs of the greasy medicine-covered, thick-layered gauze, replacing it with fresh plaintan leaves and light gauze. The fervent prayers were applied as earnestly as the live, green leafy herbal wrap. Each day Pasquale's wounds improved, and his legs and feet were saved.

If it were not for his grandmother's recalcitrance and refusal to concede medical defeat without exploring options, my father likely would have spent the rest of his life as a bilateral amputee.

When I first heard this story of my great-grandmother's stubbornness it did not surprise me or raise a question of foolish disregard for health. The narrative was an affirmation of a genetic transfer of *testadura* (hard-headedness) from Great-Grandmother Giuseppina to Grandmother Nonna, to my father, Pasquale, and eventually to me.

Testadura is fundamental to courage—a raw stubbornness that pushes past fear bare-handed.

It was not because Nonna was passive or negligent that she refused a second opinion in the life and death case of her son Pasquale. Nonna was as courageous as they come and would do whatever it took to spare her first-born. For Nonna and most people of her generation, you unequivocally obeyed whatever a physician told you. *Il dottore* was a slight step below a heavenly being and whatever he prognosticated was gospel truth, and whatever he instructed for treatment was carefully followed. A physician's word and advice was never questioned. Until her death, Nonna continued the unquestioning, dutiful patient role of her late nineteenth-early twentieth century generation.

In the twenty-first century the role of patient has evolved into one of the questioning self-advocate. Many people feel as if their doctor has only a few minutes to spend on their care because they are influenced by the medical malpractice monkey on their back, busy with the overload of patients and insurance paperwork, and worrying about medical errors. Thus, in this day and age it can appear difficult to have control over one's own health care. Yet there are substantial aspects of your own health care over which you can take charge if you believe and search for them.

With courage it is possible to:

- Recognize that in every circumstance, even if seemingly hopeless, there is an aspect of which you can take charge.
- Search for an alternative approach before conceding defeat.
- Believe and hope for curative powers of your chosen approach.

CHAPTER 14

Take Charge of Your Health: Find a Doctor Who Will Work With You

I WAS TWENTY YEARS OLD AND LIVING IN MICHIGAN WHEN I WAS DIAGNOSED with rheumatoid arthritis. The course of treatment in the early 1980s was to start off conservatively: aspirin only then wait and see what happens.

"Try 12 to 20 aspirin a day and come back in three months if not better."

Although at the time I believed myself to be pretty savvy, I did not know to complain about the mega doses of aspirin. If I did complain of the side effects—sharp stomach pain, diarrhea and ringing noise in my ears—I was dismissed with, "Those side effects are expected with high doses of aspirin."

The Midwest philosophy of arthritis treatment in the 1980s did not embrace meeting rheumatoid arthritis with aggressive medications and a multi-disciplinary approach. If the least potent aspirin regimen did not work then three to six months later the doctor suggested trying a mild, non-steroid, anti-inflammatory medication. And so went the dawdling, non-confrontational approach of treatment for my roaring disease: slowly, incrementally moving up the pyramid of arthritis drugs from least potent to more potent.

At times during the first couple of years the physicians wanted to wait six months after implementing a new drug in the event a less potent drug was taking an extra long time to show its effect. But in my case, the problem was the disease was ferocious from the onset. Every minute of every day the evil auto-immune cells viciously ate away at my joints and surrounding tissues and none of the prescribed drugs were working to slow the disease.

The time wasted during the doctor-ordered testing periods was devastatingly costly. In the first nine months alone, the disease had fiercely eaten away my precious joint linings. My knuckles were so grotesquely swollen the finger tendons that lay over them were no longer able to stretch over the added swelling expanse without tearing. Instead the tendons sought the path of least resistance, slipping off to the lateral side of each knuckle at night. As the tendon pulled off its course it often pulled the finger out of the aligned joint. Pop! The popping sound of a finger joint being dislocated from its socket, followed immediately by

shooting pain, caused me to wake in my dorm room screaming and sweating. I would jolt my upper body upright, trying to
locate the wayward finger in the dark, pulling against the pain of
the weary, over-stretched tendon in an attempt to pop the finger
bone back into its proper knuckle joint place. In the absence
of adequate suppression of joint inflammation, the excruciating
finger dislocation repeated itself at random times of the day and
night. I tried my best to keep my fingers aligned with my hand,
manually popping fingers back into place, splinting my fingers
together with popsicle sticks and wearing wrist-hand-finger
splints. But without proper immune-suppression the brutal disease won, resulting in the characteristic knobby-knuckled hands,
fingers ghoulishly pulling off to the lateral (ulnar) side of each
hand.

The mega-dose aspirin not only allowed joint damage by
failing to stop the arthritic disease process, it had detrimental
side effects. Patches of gut lining had become irritated and raw
throughout my gastrointestinal tract.

After being diagnosed while in Michigan, I decided to move
to California, in part to find better and a greater variety of medical and alternative treatments for rheumatoid arthritis. For several months I tried a California internist and alternative medicine
techniques. When the combination brought no cessation of
disease or symptoms, I had decided to seek venue with a more
aggressive treatment philosophy and cutting-edge expertise. I
switched my medical care to the renowned University of California at Los Angeles Medical Center (UCLA).

My UCLA doctor stepped up treatment and I started weekly
gold injections. The 1984 Summer Olympics were being held at
UCLA. That was the year gymnasts Mary Lou Retton and Julie
McNamara won gold medals in women's all-around and parallel
bars, and Peter Vidmar and Bart Conner took gold medals in the
pommel horse and parallel bars. Security on the UCLA campus
was tight. It was nearly impossible to enter the campus. I would

joke that I had special passes to enter the campus because I was "going for the gold at UCLA."

Hence, I had learned a lesson about the importance of choosing a physician with a philosophy and expertise appropriate for my care; a lesson learned at the expense of great physical detriment. Key cartilage, joint and connective tissue had been irreparably damaged or destroyed and my gut lining would be forevermore fussily sensitive.

Equally important was finding a physician who was supportive of my current life plan. To my great relief and delight, when after ten years I had moved from Los Angeles back to Michigan, I was referred to Dr. Timothy Laing, a rheumatologist at the University of Michigan Health System.

Dr. Laing had the complete opposite approach to the doctor-patient relationship from the physician who first diagnosed me. Shortly after beginning treatment with him in the early 1990s, I informed him that I had been accepted to law school. "... And I intend to go to law school," I told him.

I braced myself for the same negative response I received from the diagnosing doctor:

"Your disease could get a lot worse from the stress of school."

"Your disease is too debilitating for the rigors of school."

"It's not possible for you to go to school with the seriousness of your illness."

Instead, Dr. Laing smiled broadly and exclaimed, "That's great You'll make a great lawyer!"

His positive approach is a welcome surprise! I decided to push my luck and fish for support. I explained to Dr. Laing the difficulty I had encountered requesting from the law school administration a reduced, first-year class schedule. His brow wrinkled, and not knowing him well, I did not know how to read his expression.

"Who do I write or call to explain your disease process and the necessity of adequate rest?"

A second supportive response! This is fabulous! With his help I know I'll be able to finish law school!

Until this point, my experience with doctors was they could help by prescribing medication, injecting gold shots into my rump or steroids into my joints; but a doctor helping me manage my disease with a mutual goal toward helping me achieve my life aspirations? *He is exactly the health professional I need! He sees me as a person as well as a patient with feelings and dreams, and a life bigger than rheumatoid arthritis!*

Admittedly, the rheumatoid arthritis became exacerbated from inadequate rest during periods of increased studying, during the stress of exams, or from having to carry the monstrous textbooks. A popliteal cyst the size of a lemon permanently ballooned behind my left knee as a result of walking down the steps from class on a day when the elevator was not functioning and I was too proud to ask someone to carry my weighty backpack.

Dr. Laing and I discussed all these disease pathology factors. But we also talked about my striving for the goal. These discussions were about trade-offs. He was direct and strong in his opinion, whether or not it was favorable to my desire. Often his opinion was not the acquiescence I desired, and at that point it was up to me to make a final decision, fully informed. There were times I knew he did not agree with my decision to lower dosages of medications, to stall treatments or to follow a vegan diet and he forthrightly told me he disagreed. I was stubborn. He was stubborn. Even when I knew he might be frustrated with a decision I made, we both believed that central to my healing was having a life purpose. I felt his support in my goal to become an attorney and I knew he would work with my disease to the best of his ability to help me accomplish my goal.

With this total life approach to rheumatoid arthritis I made it through law school. A few weeks after graduation Dr. Laing's nurse called me at home. "Dr. Laing needs to move up the date of your appointment. He would like to see you in the rheumatology clinic next Wednesday at 8:30 a.m."

Oh brother. Now what is going on with my body?

Because of the deleterious side effects of some of the heavy-duty medications I was taking for rheumatoid arthritis and myasthenia gravis, I had monthly laboratory blood work performed and the results were sent directly to Dr. Laing's medical staff.

Maybe some negative results showed in my recent blood work. Don't borrow trouble. Do not become alarmed before you hear what he has to say.

I did not question the nurse and told her I would go to the clinic at the requested time.

I had difficulty finding a parking spot in the University of Michigan Health System parking ramp and arrived a few minutes past 8:30 the following Wednesday morning. My tardiness did not appear to matter because I had to wait after check-in before being called to the examination room. The nurse calmly called my name and weighed me in. My hands felt clammy as she took my blood pressure, the rate normal. *I'm surprised it is not sky-high.* I had been pretty calm leading up to the appointment, but sitting in the waiting room I started to become anxious. I ran through the medication contraindications and disease complications I knew of in my mind. *You feel fairly well. Then again, you have been generally fatigued. Actually, you are exhausted.* I had just self-diagnosed myself into being exhausted and chuckled at my foolishness. *Stop analyzing! Well maybe my hemoglobin had taken a dive and I am more anemic than usual. On the other hand, the stress of final exams and studying for the Bar can cause fatigue.* It was difficult to shut off the hyper-analytical portion of my mind at this point.

As I followed the nurse, everything appeared routine. Little did I know what was about to occur once I passed through the examination room door.

"SURPRISE! CONGRATULATIONS!"

I jumped in fright. Gathered around the sides and head of the examination table was Dr. Laing, his nurse practitioner, Cora Yee, and three of the clinic nurses. In the center of the examination table lay a large white-frosted sheet cake. I leaned in closer to see what the bright-blue object embedded in the thick white frosting was.

"Do you like it? asked Dr. Laing, smiling, bobbing his head up and down as if an excited child.

I was so shocked I had not yet uttered a word. I looked expressionless from him to the object on the cake and then back at him.

"It is a rubber shark! We had a heck of a time finding one. But we had to have one because now that you are a lawyer you have entered the profession also known as the 'sharks'!" Dr. Laing laughed proudly at his pun as did everyone else gathered in the room.

Dr. Laing gave a little speech, gushing proud words of admiration about how I had overcome the potential barriers of rheumatoid arthritis to graduate from law school. I cannot remember if I said anything as the cake was quickly cut and distributed so that the constantly harried staff could get back to the hectic demands of their jobs. I was dumbfounded, but I was also deeply moved. This group of people had worked to the best of their ability for years so that I could stand there on my own two feet and hold that piece of cake on my own as a lawyer.

That funny, blue rubber shark has been an office fixture in every job I have ever had. I keep it as an example of the power of support. It is also a symbol of what can be achieved by taking charge of an arduous or a seemingly hopeless situation. I am eternally grateful to all the medical professionals who have assisted me in the care of many health issues and surgeries. I am also eternally grateful to Nonna for teaching me about courage; in this instance courage to take charge of finding health professionals who fit my needs.

In this era of managed health care you may believe you do not have a choice of doctors. As a state administrative law judge, it has been my experience that most managed health plans have at least one alternative physician you may select. The key is to formally ask for an alternative physician. If your health insurance plan requires a primary care physician or gatekeeper and you requested from your primary care physician to see a specialist but were denied, you can appeal that denial. The point I am making is that it is worth the attempt to find a different doctor if you are not satisfied with your current one.

It astounds me as I hear cases in my administrative law judge's role, of people who ruminate with great angst and time about wanting a health care service, only to end up in a legal proceeding. The time and angst all could have been avoided if they had simply asked their health insurer for the service or asked in accordance to health plan procedure. It is important to know the benefits included in your insurance policy, what the procedures are for obtaining health services, and what the procedures are for appealing denials of the procedures. You should ask for and have on hand a copy of your member benefits plan. As always, write the date, name of the person speaking with you over the telephone, and what you were told or what you agreed on. Follow up with a written letter if what you agreed on is important. And *always* keep a copy of any information you send.

Let's say that you have tried all the above tips and you absolutely cannot control your choice of doctor because of your health insurance or lack of health insurance altogether. Let's also say that you are frustrated because you cannot get your current doctor to listen to you, work with you and help you. I hear from many people that their physician "only spends four minutes in the examination room with me"; "does not seem to remember the specifics of my conditions or treatment plan"; "does not take the time to discuss other medication options or side effects to prescribed medications"; and "does not take the time to physically examine my sore joints or weak muscles." For these situations I suggest the following actions:

Write out a check list of items *you wish to discuss with your physician and an identical copy of the list for the doctor. Do not hand the list to the nurse who takes prelimi- nary vital signs. When the doctor enters the room hand her the list and explain that you were hoping to address the issues. As you go through the list you or the person accompanying you can jot a short answer next to the item on the list. You may not remember every detail that was discussed with your doctor, so the list and your notes will help you remember what to ask and help you record the doctor's response. Place the list in your health folder and store it in a safe place so that you can pull it out before your follow-up appointment to refresh yourself and your doctor.*

Do your homework. *Do not assume your doctor will know all options available to you or that he will have time to adequately discuss the options with you. Go to the library, get on the Internet, or call the disease-related local association or support group. Find out what options are available and seek feedback about the options before you visit the doctor. If there are options of interest to you write them out or print them. If the options are not initially dis- cussed in your doctor visit, inquire about them before the doctor exits the room.*

Stick it out! *If you are worried the doctor will not spend sufficient time examining a problematic vestige of your body, have it unveiled, sticking out and unavoidable. After the nurse finishes taking your preliminary vital signs, ask her for a gown and sheet if necessary. Plan ahead and wear clothes that will be easy for you to maneuver and expose the problem part.*

Lezione Due: Il Malocchio (Lesson Two: The Evil Eye)

Take off your shoe and sock and have that sore red toe sticking out before the doctor enters the room. That way you are not wasting his time and you are not losing the opportunity for you to have him examine it.

Finding the right doctor and working with that doctor can foster a total life approach to living a fulfilling life despite serious chronic illness and pain.

It takes courage to:

- Be your own advocate to bring about health and obtain the best treatment for your illness.
- Realize that gathering information also gathers you power over a situation.
- Find a doctor and work with your doctor to develop a total life approach to your well-being.

CHAPTER 15

Take Charge of Your Health: Educate Yourself About Treatment Options

Similar to doing your homework before a doctor appointment, take charge of your health by seeking options you (and potentially your doctor) believe will be helpful.

From its onset in 1981, rheumatoid arthritis had been ravaging all my joints ... my ankles had been no exception including my ankles. I wore Hi-Top Freestyle Reeboks since their debut in the '80s. While the hi-top style propelled Reebok into popularity, the firm hold of the shoe's high collar lent my painful, inflamed ankles the support they needed to walk. The Velcro clasp was easier than laces for my arthritic fingers to tighten the shoe firmly around my ankles.

Even with the vigilant use of flat-heeled, ankle-supportive shoes, by 2003, I would wake in the middle of the night from the sound of my pain-wracked screams. It was obvious from how my ankles looked when I walked on them that that the bones were permanently misaligned. The bones had slipped out of joint alignment, leading to a deformity called varus deviation; my ankles looking as if they were melting into themselves, twisting the inner side toward the ground. If I tried to wiggle or bend them, the ankles barely flexed, extended or moved side-to-side, a telltale sign that significant cartilage had been destroyed.

For some unknown reason, while lying in bed in the middle of the night, the ankles suddenly seized, bone grinding against bone, nerves pinched between. The pain felt as if the mask-wearing, dagger-wielding Jason of the "Friday the 13th" horror films had slipped into my bedroom in the middle of the night and full-force plunged his knife deep into the bones and flesh of the ankle joint, then viciously pulled the blade out and jabbed again and again, and again.

Exhausted from nights of terror-induced pain and interrupted sleep, I would sometimes manage to fall into a deep slumber until the sound of my scream startled me from deep unconsciousness. In the wakening moment my body was overcome by the intensity of the pain, its brutality resulting in drenching sweat.

To step down on those shrieking ankles felt as if I was stepping onto the tip of a large knife, burning searing pain into the core of my ankle. There were many mornings when I had no idea how I would be able to withstand the pain enough to walk the twelve steps from my bedside to the bathroom.

It became increasingly difficult to walk on my ankles anywhere or at any time. I tried to conceal the pain from my coworkers, but it was difficult to disguise. The long time it took me to walk down the hall to my office was conspicuous, slowly and heavily limping, exhausted and dripping with sweat from the pain and exertion. In addition to the agony, I was worried that I would not be able to care for myself or perform my job if I did not take some kind of action to address the ankle problems.

I had been working with my rheumatologist, Dr. Laing, for about six months on a stepped-up anti-inflammatory/immune-suppression program in hopes that by reducing inflammation so also would the ankle pain reduce. I had increased the injections of Enbrel, one of the new ingenious biologic immune-suppressives. Unfortunately, the Enbrel was so good at suppressing my immune system that I was experiencing a common side effect of infection, in my case, sinusitis. I had never had sinus infections previous to Enbrel. These sinus infections were debilitating, not so much because of the facial pain, but because of the huge drain in stamina. On the higher dose level of Enbrel the sinus infections seemed to occur in two-week cycles; a four-day pressure build up to the full-blown three to four day infection, four days of relief and then back again to the build-up.

Dr. Laing and I tried a different tact. I reduced the level of Enbrel in an attempt to reduce the sinus infections, and in its place increased the milligrams of methotrexate, another immune-suppressive in the chemotherapy class of drugs. Soon after, my bimonthly blood labs showed an increase in liver enzymes, perhaps related to the increase in methotrexate. Desperate, I made an appointment to see Dr. Laing. He explained that outside of a medication regimen, the only option for the pain relief was to have my ankle fused.

"Fusion of the joints in your ankle would relieve much of the pain," Dr. Laing elaborated.

"I am barely forty. I don't want to walk stiff-footed," I protested without a bit of shame about being vain.

"Nonsense. The orthotics technicians build a mound on the outside sole of your shoes. When you take a step, you roll off the rounded part of the sole, thus diminishing the look of a stiff ankle walk." He relayed the information casually as if it were not that big of a deal.

"Rock and roll," I said jokingly, but felt deeply dismayed. *Yeah, right. This professor-type doc has no idea how many pairs of shoes I would have to have altered due to the ever shifting bones of my feet necessitating frequent change in shoe types.*

Dr. Laing referred me to an orthopedic surgeon. I had tremendous confidence in the orthopedic surgeon who had performed part of my complicated knee replacement surgeries and decided to see him. I waited over two hours until the knee surgeon entered the examination room. Apologetically, Dr. Urquhart explained that orthopedic surgeons had become highly specialized and I would need to seek a surgeon whose specialty was ankle surgery. *I took half day off work and waited all this time to be told I need to see a different kind of specialist? It's not good enough to specialize in a lower extremity; the specialties are even more localized?* The knee surgeon referred me to the leading ankle surgeon at the University of Michigan Medical Center. Before he left the examination room, Dr. Urquhart gently forewarned me that the only surgical option available would be ankle fusion.

So two specialists had forthrightly disclosed that ankle fusion was the only option, but I would not accept total fusion as an option. I was only 42 years old and I would not give in to a permanent fix that resulted in a stiff gait that made me look even more disabled, at least not until I had scoured for and pursued all options. Nonna's *testadura* was in full force.

I had to wait several weeks before the ankle surgeon had an available appointment time. During those weeks the nocturnal pain/scream/sweat occurrences were unrelenting as were the difficulties walking on my ankles.

Again, I waited several hours after my scheduled appointment time until Dr. Femino, the ankle surgeon entered the room. He held up one of my ankle X-rays so the fluorescent ceiling lights illumined from behind and he used a pen as a pointer. "You can see that in between the bones that make up the ankle and subtalar joint there is no thick opaque line. The opaque space usually indicates the presence of cartilage. The absence of a clear opaque line means that your cartilage is eroded so extensively that most of your bones have fused together."

"It is my understanding from viewing previous x-rays that the cartilage was mostly gone years ago," I noted.

"There is no longer any movement in the hind part of the ankle. But you still have a limited ability to flex your ankle. Because you have some movement I would not fuse your ankle."

For once a doctor had told me he would not fuse my ankle.

Dr. Femino was seated on a stool lowered to the same level as the chair in which I was seated. He had one of my bare feet in both hands. One hand tightly grasped the part of the ankle that attached to my leg. With the other hand he held my mid-foot. He was twisting and bending the ankle as if testing for movement. He changed hand formation and tried to rock the hind of my ankle in back and forth motions. He was very focused. Not much of the joint was moving in response to his tugging and twisting.

"I am a circumspect doctor," he stated, and I will not put an ankle replacement in you. The research shows that the current ankle prostheses are unsuccessful approximately 30 percent of the time. Because the failure rate is high, I will not perform the surgery. The bones in your ankle now have varus misalignment. In any event there will need to be a separate procedure before the replacement surgery to realign your ankle joint. After the realignment surgery you will not be able to bear weight for up to three months."

Dr. Femino continued sitting close and at eye level. I believe he saw in my eyes the crushing feeling that was sinking through my stomach. He was, after all, "the Medical Center's top ankle specialist." I had presupposed he was the answer to my increasingly debilitating predicament. Yet he was telling me he would not perform an ankle replacement. I was afraid I would start to tear up if I acknowledged the exploding inner disappointment.

Finally, Dr. Femino cut into the silence. "There is a surgeon who is highly respected. He practices in Iowa. I visited him and observed one of his surgeries. I wrote out his name and contact information for you. There is also a surgeon in Michigan, Dr. Paul Fortin, I could recommend as well if your insurance limits you to doctors in Michigan."

He handed me a piece of paper on which were the names and addresses of the two surgeons. This highly specialized ankle surgeon was technically my third consult. I continued to feel as though I had found no good options.

The next day was a particularly grueling day as I had to drive to and conduct five hearings in three cities. When I got back to the office in the evening, I had a voicemail on my office phone and a voicemail on my cell phone from the University of Michigan surgeon's office. The messages said that Dr. Femino had already called and spoken with the Iowa expert and that the Iowa surgeon's office was expecting my call.

Can you really have surgery in a state more than eight hours away? How will you get home from the surgery? How will you get to all your post-operative appointments if they are out-of-state?

My feelings of "no good options" began to conjure other negative concerns. *Had it not been only a couple of years since your fourth total knee replacement? Can you put my body through another major surgery so soon?*

Unlike knee replacement surgery where they encourage weight-bearing the day after surgery, ankle fusion or ankle replacement surgery prohibited any weight-bearing for six to twelve weeks, making it very difficult to live independently and impossible to drive. Most post-operative patients could carry some of their body weight on a walker, crutches, or cane. My wrists and elbows had eroded so significantly from rheumatoid arthritis that using those tools to become semi-mobile would not be an option. *Once again you will have to ask people to help you. How will you get to work if you can't drive and walk?*

My anxiety grew further. I realized that in addition to dreading being a bother to people, I also dreaded having another scar. I thought about the prospect of another surgery, dependence on others and the loathed scar. *Boy, what a pity party you are having. What did you utilize in the past to keep in the positive and move forward? Why can't you summon courage or see a clear path? Go within. Figure out what is bothering you.*

It took two days to figure it out. I forced myself to break the "frozen by fear" state by taking action. One of the most important steps I can take to overcome a frozen state of fear is to do something … anything … TAKE ACTION. Mutter *"Coraggio, Lisa"* under my breath and act! It need not be a grand heroic act. In this case the action was gathering as much information as I could about the surgery.

I called the Iowa surgeon's office and the staff kindly offered to fit me into whatever appointment time would fit my need. I contacted my insurance company and confirmed that my insurance policy covered the consult and surgery performed by either the Michigan or the Iowa surgeon. I researched directions to the Iowa doctor and overnight accommodations. I studied general information on ankle replacement surgery and the time and tasks involved in rehabilitation. This was sounding doable; it dawned on me that I had broken my frozen state by simply taking action and now I had armed myself with information.

In this case, information equaled power. Power produced control. I had stumbled back upon one of my vital principles: *you can always find some aspect of your life, your health and your attitude over which you have power*, and from that power you can take charge.

I had gained power by gathering information and educating myself about treatment options for my ankles. In only a matter of hours I was able to break the immobilizing, unproductive and negative feelings of fear and self-pity. That did not mean I had made my decision to have surgery, by whom and where, but I had made a decision that I would seek a consultation by the expert in Iowa and by the surgeon in the Detroit area of Michigan if need be. I would bring my X-rays and listen to what the surgeons said. At that point I would have five doctors' opinions and make a decision.

In the meantime I would seek quotes for building a ramp in my garage leading up and into the door of my home which would replace the two steps that currently existed. The ramp alone would make me independent because I could enter or exit my home via scooter. I would locate and sign-up for wheelchair transportation options to get me in my scooter to work. If I had to refrain from walking for a length of time, my plan was to open the garage door, ride my scooter down the ramp and out of the garage, onto the lift of the wheelchair van, remote-close the garage door so that no ice or snow would get on the ramp, and ride the wheelchair van until it unloaded me at the ramped handicap entrance to my work building. *Yes!*

For me, gathering information was taking charge and acting on the information garnered a feeling of control. So what had changed? Researching and working on a plan gave me the feeling that I had options and I had some control over my condition and my life. I was no longer mired in confusion, fear or hopelessness.

I thought back on Nonna and how she had taken charge in the only ways she knew: *Il Malocchio*. In times when her situation seemed hopeless, she could always find a way to take charge, even if viewing her actions from an outside perspective they appeared to be negative.

If you believe you have lost control and there is nothing left you can do, think again.

With courage it is possible to:

- Identify what part of your life, health and attitude you have power to control.

- Figure out how to manage a challenging situation in a different way.

- Keep searching or trying until you find an answer or solution.

- Keep searching until you find a treatment option that suits you.

- Acknowledge you may be immobilized by fear.

- Take an action step to break free from immobilizing fear.

CHAPTER 16
Take Charge of Your Attitude

THE INTERNAL SCRUTINY OF X-RAYS AND MRIS CONFIRMED MY SYMPTOMS; MY ankles were trashed. The many stone-shaped bones that assembled to make an ankle joint had been bereft of cartilage for years. Some of the cartilage-bare bones ground together and eventually fused the joint. Other bones grew shark tooth-shaped spurs. It was painful enough to walk on during the day, but during sleep time either my ankle bones pinched nerves between them, the razor sharp spurs mercilessly dug into the surrounding flesh, or the cartilage-bare, tender, raw bone surfaces angrily scraped against one another. Whatever was occurring physiologically, the pain was excruciating and unrelenting.

Those were disturbing and sleepless nights. I had to work very purposefully and diligently on my attitude. I had to talk myself through the incredible pain and get a grip on my thoughts and emotions so the pain would not engulf me. It was in the middle of the night, when it was dark and conducive to panic, when I was sleep-deprived and it was easier to feel sorry for myself, when there was no other human awake to call and divert my attention from overpowering pain. I did a lot of talking to myself and to God during those midnight hours, half sitting, head thrown back, body clenched in a pain-wracked grip, body shivering as my sweat-soaked skin and pajamas hit the cold night air. I had to desperately fight panic, fear and despair. I argued with myself about the attitudes to adopt as only an attorney-judge can do by herself in the middle of the night ...

> *You can wake up in the morning and believe "woe is me." You can say to yourself it is not fair you cannot go running today as passionately and obsessively as you did before having rheumatoid arthritis. You can worry that you will not get enough sleep to function at your job. You can swirl up a great brew of anxiety that you will no longer be able to perform your job ...*

Or

> *You have the ability to take charge of your thoughts right now, with haste. Be thankful that you can actually take steps to the bathroom, no matter how slow the go because of the fierce pain. Do you not remember the wheelchair days? You bargained with God that if He only allowed you to walk from your bed in the morning to the bathroom. You can choose to*

stop the panic from thinking, "I am never going to make it to work on time because the shooting pain makes it impossible to step down on my feet …" and instead utter, "Thank heaven there are only a few steps to the shower and you know you will feel better once you are in there. You alone can control your attitude right now. Falling into a peaceful inner state, wrapping yourself in warm love will prevent the demonically, powerful pain from engulfing you. Your attitude will shape your tomorrow. Come on; take a firm grasp of your attitude and pull it into the positive.

Underlying the fraught, middle-of-the-night, inner-argument was the fact that I had a choice of my emotional outlook in that moment and in the future. I could choose a positive outlook or I could choose a self-pity attitude where I felt defeated. I was the writer, director and producer of a scene to play out that moment, the coming hours, and the next day. It was up to me to choose how the script would unfold. Would the scene be uplifting or depressing? Would the story end in victory and love or finish in tragedy?

Your energy level may be limited so do not waste your valuable energy listening to your own thoughts of despair. If you allow yourself to feel less positive, you may surrender, give up.

Another important aspect to taking charge of attitude is control over with whom you choose to surround yourself. You may not be able to choose which family members or coworkers surround you, but you can choose who your friends are. Pay attention to how you feel after talking with or spending time with friends. Do you feel depressed, irritable, insecure or anxious? Do you feel drained of your joy and energy? Did the friend spend the time together complaining? Did the friend present the worst case scenario for your health situation and without an offer of solution? Did the friend elicit feelings of outrage or offense?

Some people will always feel offended and you will not disappoint them in that regard. These so called "friends" are a big drag on your ability to stay in the positive. Be wary of the misguided belief that you should feel sorry for or obligated to the person. I support helping out a person in need, but a person who is constantly dragging you down oversteps the boundaries of friendship. The person who does not respect the boundaries of friendship is not a friend, and you should be cautious to limit your contact with that person.

Initially, I try to give a person the benefit of the doubt. At times it is not easy for me to discern whether a person is acting out of love or goodness, or rather due to some other conscious or subconscious motivation. I use a quote to help me during this deliberative process. The quote was uttered by Pope John Paul II at the canonization Mass of Edith Stein, who converted from Judaism to Catholicism, became the Carmelite nun Sister Teresa Benedicta of the Cross, and died in an Auschwitz gas chamber rather than turn her back on her Jewish brethren.

Sister Teresa Benedicta of the Cross says to us all: 'Don't accept anything as truth if it is without love. And don't accept anything as love if it is without truth! One without the other is a harmful lie.'

The powerful wisdom within Pope John Paul II's quote helped me to recognize that a friend will help you out in times of need, and will respect your feelings and support your special needs. In other words, surround yourself with people who, when you think of them or see them place a smile across your face.

With courage it is possible to:

- Start each day with a positive outlook, no matter if pain plagues you or your situation seems gloomy.

- Recognize that in every circumstance you have a choice of attitude and a choice of how you will live your life through the circumstance.

- Acknowledge that your attitude will impact others positively or negatively.

- Surround yourself with people who bring joy to you, who fill you with love, who affirm your health-building actions and who support your beliefs.

CHAPTER 17

Take Charge of Thoughts and Actions Through Reframing

YOU WILL FIND IT EASY TO SURROUND YOURSELF WITH PEOPLE WHO PLACE a smile across your face if joy emanates from your heart. You will be amazed to discover the magnetic force of a joyful spirit. There may be a feeling that you have no control over the fatigue or pain from your chronic disease and therefore it is not possible to feel happy. But you do have control over whether you choose positive *thoughts,* and therefore a joyful spirit, or whether you choose negative thoughts and negative spirit. This is what I call "reframing."

No matter how wretched the situation or picture I work at placing a new frame around it. I eventually had the two ankle fusion surgeries. After each of my surgeries I was forbidden to bear weight on that fused ankle for twelve weeks. The surgeon had sawed bones and sliced off bony protrusions, realigned joints, leveled the joints with bone chips and bone glue, and had inserted plates, screws, rods and various hardware. It was absolutely critical that I not step down on the ankle for three months to allow the bones and bone chips to heal, fuse and remain aligned.

I had purchased a used electric scooter and had a ramp built in my garage. I had enrolled in the Lansing-area paratransit van program to transport me to work. The public paratransit system assigned me a pick-up time. A wheelchair van would arrive at the approximate time, lower its wheelchair lift, lift me and my scooter into the van, securely fasten the scooter and drive me to work. The program required that I be ready fifteen minutes before my scheduled time and there was no telling how many people would get picked up or dropped off while I was riding to my destination. In reality, I was at the mercy of the program, but I avoided that claustrophobic thought by reframing it to a more positive angle: I was able to return to work one month after surgery even though I would not be able to walk or drive for another two months, and it was the paratransit program that made work possible. In addition, I had the sense of being independent and simultaneously could be transported with the heavy and large scooter I needed to use at work.

Okay, that had been reframe *numero uno.* The reframe technique had been successful in the months following my first fusion surgery. Therefore, I had not expected the emotional struggle after my second surgery. The first week back to work after my second ankle surgery my pick-up for work times were changed to 6:40 a.m., even though I did not have to be at work until 8:00 a.m. That was one whole hour and twenty minutes early even though I lived only fifteen minutes from work. I had to wake an hour earlier because it took me significantly longer to get ready for work. Not being able to step down on my left foot I had to swing out of bed onto my scooter, drive the scooter into the narrow bathroom, and transfer out of the scooter onto the shower bench in my shower. After drying myself without getting too much water on the scooter, I drove from my closet with clothes on my lap, being careful not to catch a sleeve or pant leg in the wheel, and tossed the clothes on the bed so I could transfer and change lying down. *Phew!*

While my pick-up from home was earlier, my return to home rides were changed to after five p.m., meaning I arrived home after six p.m., almost 12 hours from when I left in the morning. And in the Michigan winter that meant I left in the bitter cold, pitch dark and arrived home in the bitter cold, pitch dark. In truth, I probably had not regained my stamina after surgery because previously I had worked longer hours on a consistent basis and not felt so physically exhausted or emotionally trapped.

Soon, I began to dread riding the van. I would sit and try to devise in my mind ways I could instead get into my car one-legged. *If I could just position my cast over the console I could drive myself to work. It's such a waste of time to hectically rush in the morning just to wait while driving around Lansing picking up then dropping off passengers before it's my drop-off turn.*

It was at the end of the week when I was exhausted from over-exerting myself all week that the reframe I needed came crashing down on my head. It was after 5:00 p.m.; the van had been a little late picking me up from work. As I was being loaded by the van's lift the driver informed me that we had to pick up another passenger. Through the dark I noticed that there already were two other passengers fastened by their wheelchairs in the van.

Lezione Due: Il Malocchio (Lesson Two: The Evil Eye)

Oh great. It will be at least an hour before I get home. It seemed interminable.

I started to feel anxiety and the throat-closing claustrophobic feeling of reaching an emotional limit. I was usually cheerful and chatty with the driver or passengers but my negative thoughts made my lips tense. I avoided as much eye contact as possible. I turned my scooter in the narrow space of the van's middle aisle and tried to back into the only spot available for fastening: the rear right corner. As I backed-up and passed the man fastened in the left front corner of the van I noticed he had cerebral palsy. His head was contorted to the side and fell against the neck rest of his electric wheelchair. When I maneuvered into my spot in the rear corner and was being fastened down by the driver I noticed that the elderly woman in the wheelchair in the left back corner of the van was the woman who rode the van to and from dialysis. She had looked deathly tired when I saw, her but she was cheerful and sweetly called "Good night, Honey" as she exited.

The reframe hit me. Both of these fellow passengers had a situation where they would never walk or drive again. Their means of transportation would *always* be the paratransit van. I only had to ride the van for eight weeks. *Reframe.* The sweet woman would have to ride the van several times every week to stay alive. *Reframe.* As if the universe was emphasizing the life lesson for me, the man we picked up next was a quadriplegic who necessitated a personal assistant for the most basic of needs. What a difference it made to the way I felt about the situation to view it from a different angle. I felt much lighter and it felt doable. Within the positive reframe, I recognized how my spoiled *prima donna* view had led to dissatisfaction. I tossed the diva feather boa and wrapped myself in the warmth of gratitude for all I possessed.

You can take charge of your thoughts and actions even in emotionally trying situations. The next time you find yourself feeling trapped or frustrated, stop, take a step back in your mind and try to reframe your thoughts. You may be surprised at how quickly you can go from feeling frustrated and angry with a situation to chuckling inside. And surprise again; you may find a smile on your face reflecting the newfound inner chuckle.

With courage it is possible to:

- Not allow one day to pass without recognizing a positive in your life.

- View a challenging situation in a different way.

- Reframe your thought to bring your attitude into the positive.

CHAPTER 18

Take Charge of the Aspects of Your Destiny that You Can Control

I REMAIN THOROUGHLY ASTONISHED AT THE NUMBER OF PEOPLE WHO, AFTER my diagnosis of severe rheumatoid arthritis, told me I was lucky because I could have government disability aid for the rest of my life.

"Congratulations! You do not have to work a day in your life," they exclaimed as if I had just won a lottery jackpot.

Many of these same people told me I was crazy or acted if I was crazy when instead I sought further education and employment.

They are the ones who are crazy, I thought. *What about my brains and talent? Why would I not want to utilize my intellect and intuition? Was it not part of my responsibility to share the wealth of aptitude I had been given? What about my driving ambition? Why would I not want to work?*

I may not have been able to use my body well, I may not have had control over the deleterious effects of my disease, but I did have control over whether I could have employment. And by being employed I could cover the expenses to live in a safe and handicapped-accessible home, to drive a safe and manageable car, to have benefits such as paid sick leave for doctor appointments and surgeries, and most importantly, to have sufficient health insurance. I believed securing employment was a means to take charge of the basic necessities to live, while accepting government aid would surrender control over those fundamental aspects of living.

Immediately following graduation from law school I wanted to enter a career in patent law because of my passion for and training in science. My brother consistently asserted that the most important aspect of the career for me should be good health care benefits. I accepted my first job as lawyer with a non-profit disability rights agency for a measly $27,000 per year salary. But as an agency that in part advocated for equal access to health care for people with disabilities, the job carried excellent health insurance benefits. To be honest, secretly I was somewhat frightened that I might not be able to perform the physical functions of a full-time job. But I also knew the only way I could take charge of my destiny was by *trying* to work.

Although I had successfully endured law school, I had continued to struggle with an oppressive lack of physical stamina. *Could my body truly handle working 40 hours a week, full-time job, week after week?*

As fear and doubt set in I grew anxious. After accepting the staff attorney position, I met with the dynamic executive director, explained my stamina concern and asked her if I could start at 9 a.m. instead of 8:30 a.m., as did the rest of the staff. She kindly replied that she understood my concern. I was surprised when she asked, "Why don't you try for the first few weeks to start at 8:30 a.m. If you find that you are unable to physically meet the morning start time, then let me know."

It sounded like a reasonable compromise of our individual interests and I agreed.

The weekend before my Monday start date, I laid out a week's worth of suits, underwear and shoes. I took naps on Saturday and Sunday in an attempt to stock-up on rest. *Thank you, Lord.* I made it to work each day of the first week and worked until 5 p.m. When I got home at 5:30 p.m. I ate dinner and fell directly into bed but I had succeeded! Unbeknown to me at the time, my new boss had taught me an invaluable lesson: Do not assume the worst. How do you know unless you try?

What happened next was an even more profound lesson. I discovered great fulfillment in advocating for people with disabilities. The more egregious the case the more passionate I became, and the more work I put into the case. I was now working late most nights, some weekend days and traveling around Michigan and the United States. Who would have dreamed that within just three years of graduating from law school and accepting the staff attorney position I would have traveled all over the world lecturing about the newly enacted Americans with Disabilities Act and would have co-written amicus briefs to both the Michigan Supreme Court and the United States Supreme Court?

The more impassioned I became, the more energy and stamina followed. The inexplicable, yet fantastic, power surged as incredible career and life opportunities continued to unfold, from disability rights staff attorney, to Human Services Policy Advisor to the Michigan State Senate, to Health and Human Services Policy Coordinator for Michigan Governor John Engler, and currently as a State of Michigan Administrative Law Judge. The opportunities all stemmed from the *Il Malocchio* philosophy of taking charge of the aspects of my destiny I could control. I may not have been able to control my destiny with regard to the physiological pathology of rheumatoid arthritis, but I could control the education and employment aspects of my destiny.

The invaluable life lesson I learned was that my destiny in large part had its roots in my thoughts. If my thoughts are negative and limiting, so are my actions limited and thus my destiny is limited. If my thoughts are positive, hopeful, imaginative, willing and courageous, so will my actions be hopeful, expansive, willing and courageous, and my destiny will be as full as I imagine and dare.

My friend and passionate disability-advocate RoseAnne Herzog says she believes anyone can initiate and be successful in her own business as long as she has focus, confidence and drive. In her book, *Unlikely Entrepreneurs: A Business Start-up Guide for People with Disabilities & Chronic Health Conditions*, she profiles many successful business persons and notes that each has a serious and permanent health challenge. In her consulting practice she points out that other people with less serious health challenges often fail to get over the start-up phase or fail to succeed because they remain trapped by their feelings of worthlessness and despair. RoseAnne's message is "Usually it is the individual's attitude that influences their ultimate success or failure." Taking heed of her message, I admit I have two diseases, yet I use courage to refuse any belief they are hindering disabilities, lest my thoughts grant power to disable my dreams.

With courage it is possible to:

- Believe you are the master of your destiny.
- Break free from negative, limiting thoughts so you can imagine and dare.
- Find your life's purpose and "*andiamo!*" (Go for it!)
- Believe you can succeed.

CHAPTER 19

From "*Mangia tutti!*" to "*Mangia bene!*"

Okay, I admit it. I am a foodie. I think about food all the time. I become excited when culinary morsels delight my palate. The morsels linger on my tongue, my eyes close and I tune out the world to fully experience every flavor, texture and fragrance. A low moan of "Mmmm …" begins the mantra of pleasure as enchantment moves through my body and ends with a toe-tapping code for bliss.

I cannot help it. I was raised in a family whose gatherings and interactions were centered on food. As a child, every Sunday we attended Catholic Mass at St. Gertrude Church, walked home, got into the family station wagon and drove two miles to our Italian grandparents' house. A rich garlic, tomato and parmesan cheese aroma greeted our nostrils at their driveway, the savory wafts having escaped through the front and back doors, both wedged ajar to dispense dense steam generated by a furiously boiling 10-gallon spaghetti pot.

There were always several courses to the all-afternoon meal. We always had insalata (salad). With his well-worn penknife in hand, Grandpa Francesco would stand over the oversized aluminum tub, mindlessly peeling and slicing into halves cloves of raw garlic, tossing the large chunks onto the mound of endive leaves as he told us stories in his usual jovial manner. He grabbed the gallon tin can of olive oil from its place on the counter and flung its bitter, green-gold viscous contents across the greens and garlic. When a sufficient flood of berry-colored vinegar, made from his prior year's red wine was added, Grandpa Francesco's large, calloused hands, remarkable for the long pointed fingernail on his right pinkie, would gently toss until an *insalata perfetto* (perfect salad). As a kid, my siblings and I loved Grandpa Francesco's *insalata*, stabbing forkful after forkful toward the end of our meal. But I learned to be wary of its treachery, lest my tongue be prickled by a curly endive or scorched by a fingertip-sized piece of raw garlic.

There was always *carne* (meat) or *pesce* fish at the family meal. Often, it was the carcass of an animal my grandfather, father or older brother had macho-slain: deer, rabbit, pheasant, or fish, not to mention a multitude of squirrels. As if in revenge for the damage they inflicted on Grandpa Francesco's garden, on the table the squirrels were displayed, skinned and baked, their puny legs sticking stiffly upward from the baking dish. There was an impressive variety of fresh water fish the Gigliotti men had seduced to their hooks from Lake St. Clair or the Detroit River. Oh the treat of what I called "*molto* meatballs!" (huge meatballs). Each *molto* meatball measured the size of your hand! My siblings and I would delightedly dig to discover whether the treasure of hard-boiled egg, cleverly buried by Nonna, was hidden inside the dense meatball dominating our plate. Of course our hunt proved successful! Our eyes would grow wide when Nonna's well-worn aluminum baking sheets were pulled from the oven with pork steaks piled three or four layers high. Each pork steak lusciously encrusted with rich Italian herb and parmesan cheese bread crumbs. Each bite of the luxuriously rich favorite tenderly melted into a taste-bud pleasing explosion until every layer of steaks on the baking sheet disappeared.

There was always *vino* (wine) at the family meal, the amber-pink, oak-musty wine made annually by my grandfather. Years back, Grandpa Francesco brought grapevine cuttings from his hometown in the Catanzaro region of Calabria. He lovingly coaxed the grapevines up and over the frame he built above his six-feet-by thirty-feet cement patio. The thick, rough grape leaves created a canopy to shade us in the summer during our patio meals. By late August-early September, the green-hue cast on us below seemed to cool us from the oppressive Michigan humidity. Voluptuous clusters of green to purple grapes sent forth their sweet fruity essence—a bit of heaven in this small backyard of a blue-collar Detroit suburb.

After Labor Day but before the first frost, Grandpa Francesco and Nonna fought off the invading pillager birds, squirrels, wasps and bees, and cut the succulent fruit from the vines. Nonna poured the purple globes into the ancient wood crusher as Grandpa Francesco vigorously cranked the handle until all the fruit had been mashed between the inescapable metal teeth of the crusher's gears. The deep purple slimy mash was pressed in the European wood-slatted cast iron wine press so that every bit of the mauve-colored grape juice had been extracted. Fermenting took place in deep earthen crocks in the garage or basement. After fermentation Grandpa Francesco would age the precious nectar in large oak barrels in his cool, dark wine cellar. When my siblings and I were young, we were forbidden to play in Grandpa's wine cellar, entering only if instructed to fetch a quart jar of the home-canned slimy black mushrooms shelved next to the barrels.

Every guest at Grandpa Francesco's table had at their place setting a small, thick-walled, cylindrical glass resembling those from which juice is served at greasy-egg diners. Grandpa Francesco's wine was served in those glasses at meals or at the arrival of guests. *Vino* was an integral part of the celebration and tradition of the family meal. Even as kids a small amount of wine was poured for the meal-commencing toast, raised to the cheer "*Salute!*" (to your health). Although we had *vino* at each family meal, we never abused it as children, nor have any of my siblings or parents abused alcohol as adults.

And there was always pasta at the family meal. If we were fortunate the pasta was homemade by Nonna who had spent the entire morning or prior afternoon in the laborious process. With her two bare hands she would mix the dozen eggs, cracked into the well she had dug in a mound of flour, blending and folding until the gargantuan sticky blob would accept no more flour. The springy dough was rolled into thin sheets that at times spread the width of the kitchen table. Quickly, deftly, she would then cut thin strips about one-third inch wide, the length varying with the size and shape of the rolled dough. To enter her kitchen it appeared as if a flour and noodle tornado had hit, as there was flour dusted on every horizontal kitchen surface with strands of noodles drying atop. If the counter and table tops were not sufficient, the long thin noodles were hung from broomstick dowels balanced one end on the edge of the table, the opposite end on a kitchen chair. Nonna's handmade pasta had a full egg flavor and a chewy texture into which it was satisfying to bite. Store-bought packaged pasta is completely unlike fresh pasta and it is a great injustice for fresh pasta to be categorized the same as packaged.

When I say " there was always pasta at the family meal" I am not exaggerating. Thanksgiving Day meal in America is a feast of overabundance, from the first Pilgrim and Indian celebration to modern day celebration. There are the essential feasting elements: roast turkey, stuffing, mashed potatoes, gravy, sweet potato, squash, cranberry relish and pumpkin pie, and our Thanksgiving Day table was crowded with all the essential feasting elements as well. Nonna's turkey stuffing recipe had an Italian twist of course. Her secret ingredients: browned Italian sausage pieces, slivered almonds and yellow raisins, all of which added sweetness to contrast the pungent traditional sage herb, onion and bread crumbs mixture. The turkey baked for hours and within its cavity Nonna's Italian-American ingredients married to produce the most incredible stuffing known to man. I do not make mere assertions. No mortal man has ever returned to plain stuffing once Nonna's Italian sausage stuffing passed his lips. For me, Nonna's Italian sausage stuffing, with its chunks of sausage, slivers of almond, fruit and bread, was a perfect meal unto itself.

As if Nonna's Italian sausage stuffing and all the additional Thanksgiving feasting elements were not enough food upon which to gorge ourselves, we always had the almighty huge Italian-ceramic bowl of pasta with marinara sauce squeezed into a space on the table. *Always there was pasta* at the family meal, even at Thanksgiving.

"*Mangia!*" (Eat!) was the call to commence each feast. Whether from around the kitchen door leading into the kitchen or through the screen into the backyard garden, "*Mangia!*" was the call and grandkids scampered as if starving domesticated cats to their places at Nonno's table. Nonno already was seated, always at the head of the table, his back facing the windows into the backyard garden.

Our plates were served filled to the brim and heaped two inches high, sometimes three inches at the apex of the mound, with Nonna's homemade pasta drenched in the rich, thick tomato sauce she had previously simmered for hours.

There was no such occurrence as not finishing every morsel on your plate. If you declined the call for a second serving the response was "*Mangia tutti!*" (eat everything) followed by the utterance of a short 'ehh' sound emanating from Nonna's diaphragm and more food was piled on your plate. *Why even ask the question of whether I wanted another serving?* No matter a response of "no thank you" or "I'm already full" more food landed on your plate. Even though Nonno had a modest blue-collar income earned at a ball-bearing supplier to the Detroit auto companies, there was enough food at each meal to feed the neighborhood.

All three generations of Gigliotti's would sit and talk and laugh and eat for hours. After we pushed back from the dish-laden Formica table, we moved to the living room and took our places on the couch or floor to nap, the majority of blood supply having been diverted to our overstuffed bellies. I was an adult when I realized that this ritual gathering with its intergenerational exchange of stories taught me the importance of family, courage, and love.

For me, food has always been intertwined with emotion. Now that I am an adult I wonder if non-Italians know that there is a food for every emotion. But I have been well-trained from childhood forward that whether celebration or refuge, there is an appropriate accompanying food.

To this day if *I feel melancholy* I seek a few precious gnocchi, those plump, gloriously dense potato and flour dumplings. I stare down at them in my bowl, happily bathing in marinara sauce and dotted with Gorgonzola cheese. *These coveted treasure-bombs will heal my melancholy better than a bowl of Zoloft anti-depressant pills.* Nonna's gnocchi are extraordinary; dense yet light. If you are Italian and have had the *buona fortuna* (good fortune) to have an Italian *Nonna o Zia* (grandmother or aunt) make gnocchi for you, you know what I am talking about. It takes about three of Nonna's gnocchi; the warm, soft, plump pillows slide down my gullet and completely fill the cold, lonely, melancholy void. Miraculously, the healing effects are lasting; it feels as if the potato dough-balls remain in my belly for two days, due to density of their mass.

If I need comfort, a bowl of Nonna's steaming Italian wedding soup, shrouded in freshly-grated Parmesan cheese, consolingly penetrates my soul and spirit. Eyes closed, I bend my face toward the bowl. Warm vapors nourishingly greet my skin. *Ahhh … pampered indulgence.* Continuing to press my eyes closed, I inhale the rising steam. The pungent, rich scent of broth and parmesan spoils my nostrils. I can almost see the gourmet mist swirling gently through my head, whirling down my esophagus, and unfurling in my chest to nourish the heart and spirit.

This luxury far surpasses the $100 facial I had in a trendy Sonoma, California resort salon. My friend Cheryl had driven me through lush green or grapevine-spotted hillsides near her home for a girl pampering, no males allowed, spa day. To a background of soft new age music, my face steamed with exotically organic flower petal essence and then slathered with decadently expensive imported Hungarian Vitamin C and Stonecrop extract cream. But even this upper-crust indulgence stood nothing against the facial and soul-rejuvenating bowl of Nonna's Italian wedding soup.

To maximize the comforting effect of this healing ritual, the steaming soup would be partaken in Nonna's kitchen. I do not even bother to chew the *acini di peppi* noodles; in my spoon they resemble a strand of spaghetti chopped feverishly into petite pellets. I let the large spoonful of broth, *acini di peppi*, and limp, cooked escarole, slide right down my throat. I feel the warmth of her homemade soup and the love with which she prepared it, penetrating and soothing hurts. At the same time I can see her out of the corner of my eye, at the counter, dutifully grating more cheese to dump on the tiny *acini di peppi* noodles left at the bottom of my bowl, as if believing that my favorite soup, with extra garnishing of parmesan, would make all things better for me. Nonna may not have known what to say to comfort me, but she knew exactly what to do to make me feel better.

I am more of the high-strung personality and nothing *calmed major anxiety* for me better than crunchy snacks. There is no crunchier a therapeutic tool than the biscotti cookie. The biscotti texture appears as if a dry sponge but it as hard as concrete. My sister and I learned how to make the narrow, half-moon-shaped biscotti from Nonna. The secret to its hard, crunchy texture is that the cookie is twice-baked. First Nonna baked a long, narrow, flat loaf of cookie dough on a cookie sheet. After the loaf cooled she cut the loaf into half-inch pieces, laid them on one side, and baked the slices until a slight toasty brown color appeared on the pan side. The cookies were then turned on the untoasted side until again the toasty brown color appeared.

Nonna made her biscotti with real anise seed and anise oil. As the biscotti became trendy among non-Italians, Nonna made her biscotti dough with almond pieces and almond oil or even chocolate. Because Nonna stored all flavors in the same container the licorice aroma of the anise biscotti permeated until all of Nonna's biscotti stored in the plastic, ham-shaped Tupperware container tasted of anise. But the anise prevalence never deterred me. I found my way into the old metal storage cabinet, peeled back the dilapidated plastic Tupperware top and filched the goods whenever anxiety hit its high. The desiccated sponge texture was necessary for the intended cappuccino dipping. But my biscotti skipped the cappuccino bath, instead, undipped lost a literal "hard" fought battle against my teeth. Each crumb-scattering crunch served to sooth and placate my anxious feelings.

Yes, I can compete with the best of the emotional eaters.

In 2006, I read an article about new scientific findings showing stomach to brain relationships. Reported in the *Proceedings of the National Academy of Sciences*, the findings showed a link between the stomach and the hippocampus, the brain's center for emotions. Researchers believed these findings provided new insight into the mechanisms by which people use food to soothe their emotions. *I could have simply told the researchers there was a connection and saved them a lot of work.* Interestingly, the researches also found that the frontal cortex brain circuits that are used when a person fills his/her stomach are the same brain circuits involved when a drug addict thinks about drugs. *This may explain why a foodie constantly thinks about food. But what if over-eating is not good for health? Can a foodie reconcile peace of mind, a healthy relationship with food, and a healthy body?*

Replaying Nonna's enthusiastic command of "*Mangia tutti*" in my mind fills me with glorious sentiment. At her table our bellies were over-filled with fabulously, flavorful Italian food, our hearts were filled with the joy from shared funny stories and our souls were filled with the love of family togetherness. As the onset of rheumatoid arthritis threatened to cripple me and my-asthenia gravis worked to paralyze my muscles, I contemplated what effects *mangia tutti* might have on my physical health. After contemplation, research, and a whole lot of experimentation, I realized I did not have to give up "Mangia tutti" entirely. Rather, I could change the family philosophy of "eat a lot of everything!" to "eat well." The *famiglia di Gigliotti* summons of "*Mangia tutti*" soon turned to "*Mangia bene*" (eat well).

The *famiglia di Gigliotti* could carry on tradition and revel in the love of togetherness and joy of storytelling, yet the filling of bellies could be with health-modified versions of Italian favorites and to a degree less than stuffed.

Use courage to:

- Identify emotional eating so that you can substitute non-food techniques such as meditation or positive affirmation to address an emotional need.

- Change a custom of "eat everything and enjoy even if eating to excess" to a habit of eating well and healthfully.

CHAPTER 20

Take Charge of Your Diet

MY OBSESSION WITH FOOD HAS BEEN A LIFE-LONG, LOVE-HATE AFFAIR. FOOD was my comforter. I could always count on food for an energy or mood enhancing fix. Among the Italians with whom I associated food was the center of every social setting. So I know as well as any foodie it can be really difficult to change your relationship with food.

My experience is that taking charge of your diet is an area where you have the greatest amount of control over your body, no matter what the condition of your body, and yield the most significant observable difference in how your body and brain feels.

For me, taking charge of my diet had to be a total lifestyle change. I am a food junkie. I am not sure I would have been as successful at the quick lifestyle change without my move to California where "health consciousness" was more prevalent than in the "marbled beef and potatoes" Midwest of the 1970s. I am also indebted to my mother and Nagymama who, after I moved to California, provided a support system that espoused healthful eating habits and was dedicated to my healing from arthritis.

I was fortunate in that an environment with resources and a supportive family made it simpler to go "cold turkey". For others, it may be more practical to begin with little steps by merely becoming aware to how your body reacts to food you ingest. Pay attention to how your body feels an hour or a day after eating certain foods or larger amounts of food. Has any person ever told you she or he feels "fan-*tas*-tic" an hour after eating a doughnut or corndog? It may have tasted lip-smacking good as it was being ingested and the psychological desire for the concentrated food fix was fulfilled, but the boost from the high-sugar doughnut soon sinks to the lethargy of low blood sugar. In addition the burning acid reflux is a repeated reminder of the high-fat corndog, as is the next-day bloating from its huge sodium content.

After the onset of rheumatoid arthritis I had been unwillingly conditioned in the pop-psychology theory of avoidance. For example, the day following an eat-fest of high-fat or high-sodium foods, my joints would be noticeably swollen and red, and with the redness and swelling came increased pain in my joints. I palpably learned that to avoid pain I needed to say "*arrivederci*" to cheeses, fried foods, red and fat-marbled meats, and all high-sodium foods.

At first the havoc-wreaking sodium was a stealth enemy. It took only a few next-day swollen pain events to recognize most processed food has hidden high sodium. A few more reactionary swollen joints and I became vigilant at reading sodium contents on food labels. Canned vegetable soup, low fat and packed with veggies, good choice, right? No! Hidden behind the wholesome disguise was a sodium fest. Restaurant-prepared bean soup, packed with fiber and protein, was also packed with sodium. Even boxed breakfast cereals or prepared oatmeal packets were loaded with sugar and salt.

Many of us have a work family, colleagues with whom we spend eight hours a day and with whom we share meals. Some of our favorite lunch locations were a greasy-grill, deep-frying vat pub and a Mexican food restaurant, both locations conveniently close to work. The menu at the pub had vegetables, but all were subjected to a bath in batter and deep fryer before being served. As much as I scoured the Mexican food menu, I knew the painful price I would pay for the deep-fried tortillas appetizer, or heavily cheese-blanketed, fatty beef or pork entree. The normally healthy red bean was refried in lard! Even a bowl of the house special tortilla soup was loaded with sodium. So, in order to control my diet I had to respectfully excuse myself from going out to lunch on a regular basis with co-workers.

My body felt its best when sticking to a non-red meat, low-fat protein diet with plenty of fresh steamed or baked vegetables, all unadulterated by salt and fats. As a result I learned to avoid foods that had side effects of pain. Family members and those with whom I shared meals began to subscribe to similar health-ful eating habits. It meant a lifestyle change for family members, which in turn would maintain healthy habits and attain good health for them as well.

Although I speak of a lifestyle of healthy food choices, tempta-tion is merely around the next corner's fast food restaurant or down the hall at the coworker's candy jar. One of the most imperative methods for me to protect a healthy diet is to not keep unhealthy snacks in the house. All prepared snacks are loaded with fats and salt. I remind myself that every food I put in my mouth should have bone and muscle building, immune-boosting components or it is a wasted calorie. I admit I should have more self-discipline, but in weak moments it is difficult to resist the good-tasting but bad-acting stuff. You have no idea how loudly those snacks call my name from behind cupboard doors or sealed refrigerator doors when I am stressed. If the snacks are not available within my home the call to snack goes unheeded. If it means I have to get in my car and head to fulfill a food urge chances are slim I will waste the inertia or I will talk myself out of the want before reaching the store or restaurant.

A word of caution about an unhealthy control of diet. In the first couple of years after I was diagnosed with rheumatoid arthritis I felt I no longer had any control over my body. As a novice resident of California, I sought the plethora of alternative healers and nutritionists indigenous to Southern California. Many were wise and helpful. Many told me of the detrimental effects of white sugar, white flour, and animal-based foods. Some told me my rheumatoid arthritis was caused by processed foods and meat. Others told me I could be cured, but only if I would rigidly adhere to an unwavering organic and all raw food diet.

I became increasingly paranoid about every bit of food I ate, and though difficult to admit, my paranoia developed into what I call "food-fear anorexia". The medical term "anorexia" means without appetite. My food-fear lack of appetite was different than "anorexia nervosa", the condition that a person suffers when she experiences a disillusion of herself as overweight and therefore basically starves herself by refusing to eat.

As more alternate health practitioners or concerned acquaintances flung "food is a poison" horror stories or "your arthritis was caused by your diet" criticisms my way; the more my paranoia grew, the number of foods I distrusted increased, and my weight dropped. I believed that my mother was catching on to this dangerous development and I suspected by the concerned look on her face that she told my grandmother.

To this day I am grateful for the tough-love intervention from my mother. It was a difficult confrontation for both of us. It also took a lot of research and experience for me to sort out the good and bad messages about food as it related to my health. The lesson learned? An extreme control of diet can be as dangerous and as unhealthy as an uncontrolled diet.

With chronic illness might also come chronic fatigue, lethargy, and pain. I experience a great reduction in those symptoms when I avoid carbohydrate-loaded snacks or meals, and instead support my brain and body with adequate, frequent, small-portioned, low-fat, low-salt, low-carb snacks and meals. I feel less joint and muscle pain when avoiding salt and fat. I have reduced the pain in my lower extremities because I keep to a minimum the amount of excess body weight and consequential strain on them.

With chronic illness, a change in symptoms is not necessarily rapid. Pain and symptoms seem to go on endlessly while new approaches to treatment seem to take weeks to bring relief. My compliance with a healthy diet, however, produces an almost immediate positive impact. Many people have told me their symptoms from fibromyalgia and osteoarthritis completely disappeared after earnestly cutting back on fats, sodium and excess weight.

I may have felt I had no control over how rheumatoid arthritis was affecting my body or how my body, brain and energy level felt. Diet was, and continues to be, an absolute way for me to take charge and have a prompt, significant positive impact.

With courage it is possible to:

- Take charge of your health by eating healthy foods in moderate portions.
- Take charge of your diet by reading labels and learning more about health building power foods.
- Change your lifestyle to one that supports a health-building diet.
- Seek the support of your family and coworkers to maintain your health-building diet.

CHAPTER 21

Lifestyle is a Choice Over Which You Have Control

As an administrative law judge for the Michigan Department of Community Health, on a daily basis I hear from individuals whose health is dangerously, negatively impacted by their lifestyle choices, including obesity. I am continuously confounded by the attitudes of 300- to 400-pound individuals who believe that their dire health situation—diabetes, arthritis, high blood pressure, or asthma—is not related to their obesity.

A portion of the cases that come before me are Medicaid beneficiaries who are dissatisfied by Medicaid's denial of a particular health care service they requested. Under federal law, that Medicaid beneficiary has the right to appeal the denial, which includes the right to a full evidentiary hearing before an impartial decision maker. I am one of those impartial decision makers for Medicaid beneficiaries who reside in the state of Michigan.

In one particular case, a mother appeared at the hearing appealing the denial of a request for gastric bypass for her 17-year-old daughter. The Medicaid representative testified that it had denied coverage for a gastric bypass surgery because the 17-year-old did not meet several criteria for coverage, namely, absence of obesity-related co-morbidities and failure to complete at least six months in a weight loss program. The hearing was emotional, the mother periodically crying. The Medicaid representative claimed that the 17-year-old did not have medically documented obesity related co-morbidities. The mother tearfully replied that the family doctor had told her that unless her daughter lost weight, within seven years the teenager would develop diabetes, arthritis and heart disease.

To the issue of failure to complete six months in a weight loss program the mother replied that her daughter had "tried every diet" but "none worked".

To my follow-up questioning the mother stated that there were no certificates of attendance in any of the better known programs such as Weight Watchers. But the mother wanted to inform me that the bypass surgery clinic staff told her that the surgery would "cure her daughter of food allergies". According to the mother, the teen's food allergies were so bad that her daughter could not "keep any food down". The statement about not keeping any food down was contradictory to the fact that the teen was barely over five feet tall but weighed over 200 pounds. The medical doctor witness for Medicaid stated there was no medical literature documenting bypass surgery as a cure for allergies. During the closing statements the mother tearfully pled with me to order Medicaid to pay for the surgery, thereby giving her daughter "the only chance at losing weight" and thus the only chance of avoiding "getting those terrible diseases."

The mother appeared genuinely distraught. But what deeply concerned me was that a mother would subject her teenager to an invasive surgery that has well-documented serious complications, including death, without first genuinely pursuing safe methods of weight loss. The mother was morbidly obese as well. Why would she endanger the life of her teenager instead of implementing a lifestyle change that supported good nutrition and exercise? The lifestyle change would not have to be expensive or sophisticated. Get rid of every scrap of junk food in the home. Take a family walk around the neighborhood after dinner instead of watching the television or playing video games. Discontinue the cable television or satellite dish and use the money to buy passes to the community recreation center or the high school pool when Midwest winters posed a problem to walking, riding bikes or other outside activities.

Perhaps you believe the situation is more complicated than my solutions pose. Perhaps the mother did not have the sophistication to know about a lifestyle of good nutrition and exercise. If that was true then I have even greater concern about the gastric bypass surgery staff who encouraged surgery instead of sending a nutrition and exercise counselor into the home to educate the entire family. Instead, the staff of the bypass surgery business filled a mother and daughter with a quick and easy weight loss promise and the false hope of a cure for food allergies, a cure claim unsupported by any reputable medical literature.

An additional disappointment was that the mother had insisted that her daughter be present at the hearing. I could not help but think of the negative psychological effects the daughter may have experienced when listening to her mother, the Medicaid representative and the Medicaid representative's physician witness talk about her being morbidly obese, bound for awful diseases and that her only hope was a convenient and quick surgery, free if paid for by the government Medicaid program.

Lezione Due: Il Malocchio (Lesson Two: The Evil Eye)

In 2005, the *American Journal of Preventative Medicine* published the results of a study showing that people having a body mass index even slightly higher than the healthy level was three times more likely to damage the cartilage in their knees, requiring corrective surgery. That same year the Canadian Institute for Health Information (CIHI) published a report with similar finding. Interestingly, when CIHI made statistical adjustments for age and gender, the figures showed that people who were overweight were *three times* more likely to get knee and hip replacements than people with healthy weights. An Associated Press article relating the *Journal of Preventative Medicine* findings ended with what I believe is an alarming quote from Dr. George Mensah, Acting Director of the National Center for Chronic Disease Prevention and Health Promotion: "Despite the increase in awareness of obesity-related ailments," Mensah said "few are taking heed" and noted 16 percent of American children, ages 6-19, are overweight. "The epidemic has no signs at all of slowing."

Dr. Mensah's message is alarming to me because it says that, even though there is public awareness that obesity can cause joint destruction, diabetes and heart disease, people are continuing to eat themselves into physically destructive, life-threatening situations at an epidemic pace. And from my experience as an administrative law judge deciding medical-related cases, I can tell you Dr. Mensah's message is not overstated. Each day I see or hear people noticeably distraught over what obesity is doing to *me*, but blatantly making no connection or taking any responsibility that the *me* is causing the obesity that in turn causes dire health consequences.

I had a series of men and women who appeared in front of me to appeal the denial of Medicaid funds to pay for gastric bypass surgery. They spoke with angry or sob-laden tones, telling me that their doctor told them if they did not lose weight they would soon experience life-threatening disease complications such as diabetes, hypertension, apnea, cardiovascular disease and osteoarthritis. What I found remarkable when listening to these people is that each spoke with self-pity and blamed God or Medicaid for their potential health consequence. "Why would God want me to have heart disease that will kill me?" "Medicaid is discriminating against me by not paying for the stomach surgery, and because it's refusing I am going to have diabetes. That's just not fair!"

I also heard the appeals of several individuals who had been denied Medicaid funds to pay for an electric scooter or wheelchairs. For all of these individuals, their stated underlying medical need for the electric scooter was obesity. They were all of working age but were on state and federal taxpayer-paid disability payments because of a diagnosis of obesity. *When did obesity become an irreversible illness that could be deemed as the basis for permanent disability payments?* The same public disability payments bought the food they overate. *But wasn't obesity a symptom of overeating, not an incurable disease?*

As harsh as it sounds, I do not believe my reflections are based on ignorance or simplicity. I myself had to overcome learned patterns of eating in order to make successful healthy lifestyle changes. Growing up, I believed every family's cookware consisted of a 10-gallon pasta pot left on the stove and reused the next day. I only knew Italian ceramic serving bowls that were large enough to bathe your newborn child for the first six months of life. I thought it was the norm to have a second full kitchen, including stove, refrigerator, sink and dining table, in the basement of your home.

I try to practice what I preach and do not bring junk food in my house. If snack crackers, tortilla chips, cookies or ice cream were present, some type of rationalization would likely permit them to find their way down my gullet. No matter if I would lock the delectables in the cupboard, freezer, or even the trunk of my car, their voices would call out to me in a plea so desperate to be eaten that I would have to comply.

I have a choice of whether to bring tasty, time-saving, processed foods into my home. If temptation is not present, I do not have to battle against its call. Despite living in Michigan with its short crop season, I try to have vitamin- and mineral-rich fruits and vegetables present for meals as well as snacks.

I do not typically watch television or DVD movies. My exercise bike, exercise ball and thigh-master block my television. If I want to treat myself to viewing one of my favorite history or political talk shows, the trade-off is hopping onto an exercise equipment item during viewing. It is a lifestyle decision I make.

Despite what the not-my-responsibility society leads you to believe, lifestyle is a choice over which *you* have control. I have a choice of what foods I put into my body, whether I exercise, and how much sleep I get and I am the master in control of those choices. The choices I make will determine whether my lifestyle will support a healthy me. I can work toward a healthy me even if I have two serious chronic illnesses by avoiding behaviors that lead to an exacerbation of those illnesses.

Use courage to:

- Choose and maintain a healthy lifestyle.
- Change your lifestyle by banning all junk food from your home.
- Change your lifestyle by substituting watching television with exercise or sleep.
- Accept responsibility for your diet, your weight and the amount of exercise and sleep you get each day.

CHAPTER 22

Take Charge of Your Health: Exercise, Body Weight and Muscle Tone

AT TIMES I FELT POWERLESS OVER THE CURRENT STATE OF MY BODY, BRAIN and energy level. As unlikely as it sounds, it was exercise, moving that same uncooperative body that helped to conquer feelings of helplessness, to take charge and to achieve a noticeable positive impact on my body and feelings.

I was one of those people who *liked* to exercise. Before my body was attacked by rheumatoid arthritis exercise was a significant part of my life. A day was not complete without some kind of workout. As a teen I ran everyday. Even if I had stayed up after midnight studying for an exam, I did not sleep before hitting the bubblegum pink shag carpet of my bedroom floor for sets of sit-ups. In part, daily exercise was a means of weight control; it helped with my indulgences in the caloric-laden Italian delectables. It was also an important aspect of emotional health. There was nothing better to clear my mind and soul than a several miles run; I could sense the unraveling of inner tumult with each padded stride and labored exhalation.

The onset of rheumatoid arthritis forced an inability to run and with it a fear that I would gain weight and muscle tone would be lost. In addition I was concerned about the loss of my proven method for maintaining mental health.

Aspects for exercise, weight control, and muscle tone are controlled by your own choice. Your body may impose limitations but I believe there are many options over which you have power. The key is you have to want to make a positive impact and make an effort toward impact. You can choose to take charge, even incremental steps toward healthy cardiovascular system, weight, muscle and mind; or you can choose to make excuses and surrender control.

Exercise. I can make a better excuse than anyone to not exercise: a double-whammy "arthritis plus myasthenia gravis" conundrum. For rheumatoid arthritis it is important to exercise and keep joints moving so they do not become stiff. Yet, too much wear and tear on an arthritic joint can cause inflammation and joint deterioration. If that is not enough of a balancing act, with myasthenia gravis too much exercise at a time can fatigue the muscle to the point of collapse.

I could be well justified to claim that exercise is contraindicated for my illnesses. Better yet, I could argue there is no exercise I could perform. Baloney! Never will you hear those excuses come from my mouth. Instead I say, "Take charge!" I believe that no matter the condition of your body, you can always find an activity that moves muscles, even if it is merely sitting or lying flat and tightening the different muscle groups in your body.

I had to be creative to find exercise that worked for me; some were born of necessity. In the summer of 1998, I had been standing at my sister-in-law Nancy's kitchen sink helping clean up after a big Italian family feast when suddenly—*crack! snap! pop!*— a series of bone-splitting crunches tore through my feet. As if by some demonic design, hairline fractures had spider-webbed through the small bones of my feet. *Why did this happen? I was only standing sink-side. No heavy-footed walking. No strenuous torque. How could mildly named hairline fractures cause such debilitating pain?*

The following summer I attended a friend's baby shower. When I stood I heard a loud "*snap*" Bone-cracking pain shot from the narrow bone on the lateral side of my right foot, through my body, ricocheting to the brain. The "*snap*" was loud enough to draw the attention of several friends to my face, which went immediately pale and beaded with sweat. *Not again! Oh please, God, I know the pain of cracked bones within my body, but don't let it be true...I don't have the time or energy, or ability to stay off my feet for the great length of time it takes for foot bones to heal!*

On both foot bone fracture occasions I only weighed 115 pounds. The bones were not breaking under the duress of excessive weight. The fractures did not occur as a result of physical duress. *So what is causing the fractures?* Although I was only in my late 30s a bone density scan revealed osteoporosis to the extent of that typically seen in an 80-year-old woman.

There is no quick fix for broken feet bones, especially mine, brittled by rheumatoid arthritis. If I was prescribed a foot cast, the bulky cast threw off my body's natural balance and irritated my artificial knee until my knee swelled. Neither my doctor nor I wanted to jeopardize the artificial knees. The only sure method for healing the bones in my feet was to stay off of them as much as possible. But my job involved walking from the Senate office building to the Capitol.

After the second round of foot breakage I told myself that instead of letting it happen again, I would be proactive and aggressively fight the further progression of bone loss and breakage.

The media is saturated with information about the ability of increasing bone density through exercise, especially bone-jarring exercise. I was not able to walk more than short distances, yet I needed a way to signal my body to keep strengthening bones.

The unfortunate foot breaking actually started my dedication to swimming. I was able to walk in water because water supported the weight of my body enough not to damage my ankles and artificial knees. My elbows and shoulders had significant arthritic limitations and were prone to inflammation if exerted. My ankles were fused. Between the arm and ankle limitations I could not swim in the normal free-stroke manner. Yet, I knew that swimming would be my greatest hope for a good cardiovascular workout. I discovered a floatation device that strapped around my waist wherein I was able to keep my head above water. I floated to the deep area of the pool and treaded water for as long as I could. *What a strenuous workout! And I did not even break a sweat!*

There are excuses for avoiding swimming. When I talked about water as an exercise aid or when I listened as a judge to individuals who claimed there is no exercise to help them lose weight, I heard a lot of "I can't swim", "A pool is difficult to access", and "Fitness clubs are too expensive to afford".

My experience does not agree with the reasons behind those arguments. I have found high school pools and community pools that are open for public use and charge anywhere from $2.00 to $4.00 per swim. Most of the public pools have steps or other accessible means of water entry. The individuals arguing they cannot afford to swim may have a cable television payment that is greater than the cost to swim two to three times per week. Sitting in front of the television will not help to maintain fitness and strengthen bones. It is a matter of *choice* on how to spend time and finances, rather than actual affordability and accessibility to exercise.

I live in the frigid Midwest. In the short distance from the community pool door to my car door my hair freezes into a shiny black ice helmet. My geographic location makes it more difficult to access a pool than my friends who live in warmer, year-round, pool-friendly climates. But it is not impossible to access a pool if I am determined. I have an impressive arsenal of excuses and it is my choice whether to use them.

To exercise or not to exercise is a choice.

Keep weight down. The importance of maintaining a normal weight cannot be overstated. For an individual with joint disease such as mine it is critical. Each extra pound I carry equals 60 extra pounds of force on my knee joint grinding against the precious tender cartilage that cushions my knee joint as I bend it to go down a step; 60 extra pounds of force grinding against the precious tender cartilage cushioning my hip joint with each step I take. The 60 extra pounds of force is compounded each time I add a pound to my body weight. Can you imagine the devastating forces if I gained 10 pounds?

Here is an alternate way to think about the negative impact of each unneeded pound of gained weight. A gallon of milk weighs approximately 8.62 pounds. At the time of my diagnosis at age 20, I was 15 pounds overweight. When I think back on it from this perspective, I was carrying two gallons of milk around my neck everywhere I went, all through the day and night, everyday. Each step I took had two heavy gallons of added weight that needed to be supported by the inflamed and tender tissues of my hip, knee, and ankle joints. I ran everyday with the added distressing weight crushing the weight-bearing hips, knees and ankles.

My first knee surgeon was blunt and gruff about weight control. He would open the door of the examination room, look at my chart, glance at me, and sternly ask, "Have you gained any weight?"

As a woman who was overweight as an adolescent I am very sensitive about being asked about my weight. Although somewhat offended, I knew I could not fathom the sheer physical devastation my surgeon saw each day in that most people had brought their own physical destruction upon themselves. He felt utter dismay at the number of joint linings he found ground to shredded pieces merely from the stress of self-added body weight.

This surgeon was a sought-after expert. He told me that as a policy he refused to replace joints of those people who were obese. He told many individuals to come back after they had lost 100 pounds. He explained to me the fervor behind his policy. On one occasion he made an exception for a 300-plus-pound man who had pled to the point of tears for a knee replacement. The man returned one week after being discharged from the time and resource-expending replacement surgery. His weight had bent backward and snapped the metal and plastic knee prosthesis. After that, the knee surgeon vowed never again to replace a lower extremity joint on a person with morbid obesity.

The truth is that obesity and obesity-related co-morbidities are the result of actions individuals do to themselves. They have control over what they eat and whether they exercise. What if I asked you to carry four full milk cartons all day? Wouldn't you try to get out of the task, expecting to be exhausted with sore knees and feet by the end of one day? Yet, that is what we ask of our bodies if we are 25 pounds overweight.

Tone those muscles. As much as "move it and <u>lube</u> it" is the motto for joint health, "move it or <u>lose</u> it" is the motto for muscle toning. There is a lot of muscle wasting that can occur with autoimmune diseases. While muscle wasting can be due to the disease process itself, a reluctance to move body parts that are sore or weak can also lead to muscle wasting. Lack of motivation to exercise can coexist with a lack of energy. The good news is that there are means of keeping muscle tone without moving body parts or with minimal movement. These means of toning muscle also utilize minimal energy.

Being from the Midwest, having only heard of yoga, I was skeptical of the claim that I could tone any muscle by merely sitting in one position. I also had a difficult time imagining how I could sit with my arthritic legs contorted into a pretzel position. I was willing to try anything that would help muscle tone so I thought to check it out.

Key to making yoga work for me was finding an instructor knowledgeable and willing to help me adapt to positions that would fit my physical limitations. For example, when the yoga routine changed to the arched-back cat position the instructor either helped me devise a similar position from a seated position, or she suggested I continue with the previous position until the routine moved to the next to pose.

I also bought a basic level yoga routine video for home use. Taking cues from the adaptations learned in my yoga class I performed most of the video yoga routine from a chair in my living room. The beauty of living room yoga is that I could wear clothing that was comfortable, I did not have to drive and walk to a class, or drag equipment—all important aspects of good joint protection.

The use of breathing techniques to release stress and bring inner peace had the bonus of helping the myasthenia gravis-related breathing issues. Within a short amount of time I noticed how the tone of my arm, leg and breathing musculature had improved from this seemingly effortless routine.

More recent studies show if you are unable to do bone-jarring exercise as means of increasing and maintaining bone density, moving muscle alone can help. Researchers believe that the bone tissue picks up signals from the active muscle. I liken it to an analogy where the bone-forming commander says to the bone-producing troops, "Hey, these muscle guys keep going at it. We had better make sure we are strong enough to handle them!"

Lezione Due: Il Malocchio (Lesson Two: The Evil Eye)

Before each of my eight knee and ankle surgeries, I planned my pre-surgery exercise strategy as if I had been preparing for an Olympic competition. I worked to strengthen the muscle groups I thought I might need after I had surgery. I knew I would need to rely on my core body muscles—the muscles of my stomach, back, and torso—to pull myself up in the hospital bed and to transfer from one surface to another without the help of my legs. I also knew my deteriorated wrist, elbow and shoulder joints would not be able to make up for immobilized legs. Most of the muscle strengthening exercises I did lying on my back in my bed, slowly raising, holding and lowering limbs. After only a few days and simple moves, the core muscles were on their way to being prepared for the post-operative competition.

As soon after surgery as my surgeon gave me the go-ahead to do light, non-strenuous exercises I would lie flat on my back in the hospital bed and lift, hold and lower the non-surgical leg. I did not want to lose any muscle tone or strength, and the movement helped me be less groggy and start to regain appetite.

Key to sustaining a healthy weight and functioning body is following a healthy lifestyle that includes exercise and linking with loved ones who join in your exercise lifestyle. Exercise that is convenient and enjoyable is more likely to be part of a lifestyle routine. Many people link with an exercise buddy, take walks with their spouse, or ride bikes with their children. For me, exercising at home with inexpensive body bands and an exercise ball works. To combat boredom I alternate among exercise DVDs. To add a fun factor I listen to motivational messages, sing along with motivating music or listen to books on CD.

As any person experienced with myasthenia gravis knows, fatigue of the respiratory muscles can result in intubation and placement on a respirator. My key to keeping respiratory muscle tone? Singing! I joined a small contemporary music group at my church. I know my lungs will receive at least one hour of deep breathing and sustained exhalation each Wednesday night practice and more than an hour on Sunday. Again, for me, exercise with a fun factor! I give great concerts while driving in my car or in the shower, all with a dual purpose of respiratory muscle strengthening so the muscles are primed in the event of a myasthenic set back.

Exercise is critical to keeping all my body parts—the parts affected by rheumatoid arthritis and myasthenia gravis and the parts not affected—primed and functioning as best that I can control. The blood-pumping endorphin high, and motivational music and messages, have the added benefit of cultivating a happy spirit!

It takes courage to:

- Acknowledge that extra weight and lack of exercise adds to a disease's detriment.
- Exercise when your body feels sore.
- Exercise when you feel emotionally or physically fatigued.
- Make a lifestyle change that includes regular exercise.
- Keep trying until you find an exercise routine you enjoy.
- Recognize that exercise is a choice over which you have control.

CHAPTER 23

Focus on the Positive to Accomplish Lifestyle Change

I KNOW CHANGE CAN BE DIFFICULT. WHEN NONNA WAS IN HER LATE 70s she was hospitalized after months of diarrhea, nausea and weight loss left her perilously weak. She was diagnosed with celiac sprue disease, her body unable to tolerate wheat or corn glutens. Her doctor told her that if she did not change her diet to eliminate all wheat and corn products she would be dead within two months.

At first, Nonna was perplexed at how to make a lifestyle change. She had spent a lifetime with *"basta"* (pasta), *pane* (bread) and *polenta* (corn mush) as her staples. She was set in almost eight decades of her Old Country ways. How could she possibly change? Her family was there to support her, reading everything we could about the disease. It was important to provide Nonna with formats that worked for her. We drew a large-print basic chart that showed the absolute no-no's in her diet. We discovered celiac sprue diet cookbooks. The most successful format for Nonna? Recipes for foods she could eat and for foods she was familiar with and she liked.

In her courageous, stubborn, *testadura* way, she made up her mind that she *could* change and *could* continue to live. Always one to choose the positive, she focused on all the foods she could eat, instead of food she could not eat. There were the Italian pole beans from her garden. Fixed with potatoes and made succulent with fresh basil and fresh garlic, also from her garden. Not a trace of wheat or corn. She often made her own version of *pasta fagioli zuppa (bean soup)* and said it was so rich with beans and vegetables she did not miss the pasta.

The point here is that an unsophisticated, stubborn, old Italian woman could make a tremendous lifestyle change for her health and healing. Did she want to? No. Was it easy for her? Not at first. But once she was handed the tools and she made up her mind to change she never went back. *Sua tutti famiglia* (her entire family)—son, daughter-in law, grandsons, grandson-in-law, granddaughters and granddaughter-in-law was there to support her. Her family would scour grocery, Asian food and health food store shelves to bring her the latest gluten-free pastas or surprise her with new gluten-free cakes and cookies.

Nonna's courage to make and stick to a drastic dietary change also taught me to focus on *tutti mangiare* (all you could eat) instead of focusing on what you could not eat. Her courageous attitude avoided self-pity or binge-conducive resentment. Nonna's ever-present emphasis on the positive provided a life-saving and mental health-saving example.

When I entered the nursing home in my early twenties, I lost weight and was dehydrated. The severity of myasthenia gravis weakened my facial and throat muscles to the point I could not chew or swallow properly. Dinner was served to me in the nursing home bed, on a bed tray over my lap. I uncovered the plate each day with the anticipation of "food, glorious food!" only to discover the same thing as the day before: three or fours globs of pureed matter. The grey glob was usually macerated cooked meat; the white mound, reconstituted dehydrated potato-flakes; the smooth orange mass, maybe carrots, possibly squash; the pulpy green pool, blended vegetation, sometimes undistinguishable. I never figured out whether they pureed my food because of my facial muscle weakness or because puree *du jour* was standard fare. Though from what I witnessed every other resident's meal was pureed, making it easier to feed those with dementia.

I could not complain because at least it was food that would pass my palate. My roommate was solely fed liquid drained via a tube inserted into the jejunum portion of her intestines. I needed be grateful that I could at least place the globs in my mouth, even if the texture was mush and the taste was not savory, and that I could spoon the mush into my own mouth, even though the dialysis wounds—one in the right arm for blood exiting my body to the pheresis machine and one in the left arm for the filtered blood returning to my body, and the compression bandages that prevented the vessel entry and exit punctures from bleeding— made it painful to bend and lift a spoon to my mouth. And I needed be grateful that I was cognizant that I was eating, unlike my cohabitants with dementia or those in a coma.

Nonna's courage to adapt to a drastic dietary change taught me to focus on all the possibilities available during a necessitated lifestyle change. Her ever-present emphasis on the positive kept her moving forward each day, embracing with exuberance aspects of the day she enjoyed. To focus on the limitations that brought about her lifestyle change would have frozen her in a bitter, resentful mood, blinding her to the pleasurable opportunities before her.

Use courage to:

- Broaden your knowledge of the possibilities associated with a new lifestyle.

- Focus on the possibilities to transform your view of a lifestyle change into positive.

- Adopt the positive view of lifestyle change into your daily routine.

- Surround yourself by loved ones who support your lifestyle change.

CHAPTER 24

Buona Notte! Take Charge of the Aspects of Sleep that You Can Control

YOU MAY NOT BE ABLE TO CONTROL YOUR QUALITY OF SLEEP IF IT IS INTERRUPTED by pain, but there are aspects of sleep that you can control. Sleep is important for a strong immune system and health-building bodies, for a positive attitude and to fight self-pity or feeling down. All the tricks that doctors recommend to improve sleep apply here. In addition, more sleep may be required for bodies with chronic illness or bodies undergoing certain medical treatments.

Do not feel ashamed to say you need nine hours of sleep per 24 hours. Set boundaries. Tell family and friends that your bedtime is 9:00 p.m. and that your alarm is set for 6:00 a.m., and ask them to respect this important healing time by calling at other times. Take charge to protect your sleep time!.

Here are additional sleep hygiene practices over which you have control:

- A regular bedtime and wake time is crucial.

- Regular exercise, except for immediately preceding bedtime.

- Stimulants should be avoided or banned after noon. Most people believe avoiding stimulants means no coffee or cola. But hidden stimulants can be steroids/prednisone (I take my full dose of prednisone as soon as I get up in the morning rather than in the evening), chocolate, tea, soda (even orange-flavored pop may be loaded with caffeine). The old-fashioned comfort tool of a cup of hot cocoa or tea before bed is also a whopping dose of caffeine that can be the cause of insomnia. Ask your doctor, nurse, or pharmacist, or read the package insert to determine if any of your medications cause insomnia and follow-up by asking what can be done to counter the side effects.

- It is a myth that alcohol can help you sleep. While alcohol may help you to fall asleep, it can cause middle-of-the-night insomnia.

- Take work out of your bedroom. It was difficult for me to break the habit of bringing work into bed. While I thought the accomplished work task would help me feel productive and relaxed, the opposite occurred; my brain was stimulated and had a difficult time settling into sleep. If possible, take your computer or work desk out of your bedroom. Even watching television can stimulate the brain. I have never regretted removing the television from my bedroom. Make your bedroom your safe haven of rest and healing. Your bedroom should only be used for sleep so that your brain is signaled "*ahhhh ... this is my resting place*" when you enter that room.

- Take your pet out of your bedroom. I constantly hear people talk about being exhausted during the day because "my dog thrashed about in my bed during the night" or "my cat kept me awake by crying throughout the night." I am an animal lover, too. All I am saying is to love your pet in a way that doesn't rob you of one of your most critical healing sources.

- Turn off the brain in whatever manner works for you. Since childhood I struggled with turning off my mind in order to sleep. I know how difficult it can be. Try to figure out what works for you. Some people meditate and fall off into peaceful sleep. Meditation before sleep does not work for me. Instead, when I lose meditative focus I become irritated and awake. Some people fall asleep to the television, radio or music. I try to do a little routine. I read a short, daily inspiration and reflect on how the message applies to me. I talk to God and thank Him for the day, and I ask for Divine assistance throughout the night.

Even if you have pain or illness, you have control over activities that can foster restful, healing slumber or thwart restful sleep. Grab the courage to toss the diet coke and banish the television from the bedroom; then grab pillows, comforter, healthy sleep habits and "*buona notte!*"

It takes courage to:
- Ask others to respect your eight to ten hours uninterrupted sleep regimen.
- Identify and take control of activities that thwart restful sleep, such as caffeine, television, and irregular sleep schedule.

CHAPTER 25

Take Charge of Non-Traditional Healing Opportunities

THERE IS LITTLE DOUBT I COULD BUY A CAR OR A HOUSE IN MY MIDWEST environs with the amount of money I have spent on alternative healing methods. Although I have never been "cured" by any of the alternative healing offerings, I do not consider one dollar or one minute spent as a waste. For me, alternative medical approaches are an area over which I can take charge of non-traditional aspects of my healing.

In addition to the traditional medical model approach to treating illness, I have explored many alternative medical offerings. I need to clarify that what I am suggesting is a balance of traditional medical treatment with an alternative medicine approach. Many of the alternative medical therapies will not harm you. But if you abruptly stop taking prescribed medication when you begin adopting alternative treatment you could harm yourself. I know from my own experience about slamming against a wall of acute exacerbation after abruptly terminating all medications in pursuit of a natural remedy.

This harsh lesson occurred only a few of years after I had been diagnosed with rheumatoid arthritis. The medical approach pharmaceuticals were not abating the disease and instead had detrimental side effects. Without adequate suppression the rheumatoid arthritis had mercilessly eaten away a great portion of my joint lining. The healthy, smooth cartilage essential to smooth, painless movement of the knee joint was decrepit and I was barely able to bend my knees or walk.

I was desperate for a cure and my mother and Hungarian grandmother were desperate to find a cure for me. My grandmother took a loan against her modular home to pay for extended treatment at an alternative medicine cancer clinic in Mexico. My mother packed the car with my wheelchair and a week's worth of belongings and drove me to the clinic, just outside of Tijuana. My mother talked to me on the drive from Los Angeles to Tijuana, trying to bolster my resolve for what lay ahead of me.

Dr. Max Gershon had escaped Nazi Germany and reestablished himself as a physician in the United States. He believed that cancer resulted when the body no longer had normal metabolism due to long-term poor nutrition and pollutant exposure. Dr. Gershon's theory for healing cancer was to detoxify the liver, pancreas and immune system for a long enough period of time that these body systems could regain normal functionality. The detoxification involved frequent coffee enemas. The body then was replenished with freshly squeezed carrot juice into which was stirred ground raw liver. The enzymes in the carrot juice would act as antioxidants, chasing any remaining free radicals in the body. The raw liver juice was to support my liver functioning. I would also have to inject myself with Vitamin B-12 as a means of providing physiological support.

Dr. Gershon's belief was that the chemicals from the prescribed medications I had taken had caused liver toxicity. His healing regiment called for the overtaxed liver to be free from chemicals, including medications. As my mother drove, we talked about the pros and cons of discontinuing all my medicines. On the one hand, the medications did not seem to be working; my joints were being ferociously eaten with no pharmaceutical medicine able to hold the demise in abeyance. In addition, one week at the clinic cost several thousand dollars, which was all we could afford. This cure-seeking trip was a huge financial burden on my grandmother and mother, so I *had* to give whatever it took to succeed.

From my years of studying physiology and biochemistry, it made sense to me that a liver could become over-taxed by the constant metabolizing of chemical agents. On the other hand, there did not appear to be any good arguments against halting the pharmaceuticals. No physical harm could come from enemas and raw juices, so I decided to discontinue my medications.

Upon arrival at the cancer clinic we met with Charlotte Gerson, Dr. Gerson's daughter, who held the personal mission of keeping her father's work alive. Ms. Gerson explained that the same principle of cancer-causing toxicity was applied to autoimmune diseases such as rheumatoid arthritis. She reemphasized the need to discontinue ingesting any toxins, such as medication, while vigorously trying to detoxify and rebuild the body. As one can imagine, it was an intense and rigorous week, and my mother encouraged me every minute of each day.

Lezione Due: Il Malocchio (Lesson Two: The Evil Eye)

At the end of the week as my mother was driving us home, I told her I thought I felt better. I still could not walk and needed to use a wheelchair, but the pain did not seem as intense. I would need to continue the daily enemas and hourly fresh juices for several months, and it would take all three of us to help continue the healing regimen. Maybe we could get friends to help, too. But if it meant I could be cured it was worth it. But, what I did not know, was that in the next several weeks the rheumatoid arthritis would flare to such an extent that my arms, legs, neck and jaw would lock-up, and acute, searing pain would result at the slightest attempt to move from my fixed fetal position.

I did not want to admit that the exacerbation may have been caused by going cold turkey from my arthritis medications. I had read that an exacerbation of symptoms could be part of the alternative medicine healing process; it could even be an indicator that the alternative method was working. How could I know whether the hope-driven alternative approach was helping or harming?

More than a year of dutiful adherence to the Gerson regimen passed and no cure. I had not even taken one step on my own feet.

In acute and entirely immobilizing pain, the deaths of my mother and grandmother deleting the help needed to effectuate the daily onerous fresh juice and enema routine, I eventually went back to taking my traditional medications while continuing an alternative healing approach.

The lapse in prescribed medications permitted the relentless disease to take a ferocious, destructive siege on my body and it took a long time to regain even a small degree of control over the disease process. But my cold turkey experience did not dissuade me from trying other alternative healing avenues, but rather, use alternative methods in conjunction with the medical model approach and consult my physician on any questionable treatments. For me, trying additional approaches focused my mind on positive healing and, as such, brought hope.

California is an abundant haven of alternative medicine. The list of alternative medicine approaches, most of which I have tried, include acupuncture, acupressure, Aryuveda, high-colonics, chi quong, Reiki, reflexology, metaphysical entreaties, rebirthing, and laying-of-hands.

On a regular basis people approach me to recommend a dietary or nutritional approach. I appreciate the well-intentioned advice from others. *You won't know unless you try it. Even if it does not bring about a cure, it may bring health to another realm.* Whatever the natural treatment approach, be it wheat grass, vitamins, mineral supplements, herbal supplements, nutritional drink mixes, chicken cartilage, shark cartilage, vegan shell powder, fresh squeezed juices, chelation therapy, or eucalyptus oil, as long as it has someone's claim to cure, and is not harmful I'll consider giving it a try.

In the process of trying I am taking control of my health by a yet unknown, acclaimed healing source. And with the thought of potential healing I have hope.

With courage you can:
- Find hope in seeking alternative healing practices.
- Find the optimal balance between the medical model and alternative treatments.

CHAPTER 26

Deal With What I am Able and "Ciao"... Let Go of the Rest

FUNDAMENTAL TO MY "TAKE CHARGE OF WHAT I CAN CONTROL" PHILOSOPHY is to deal with what I can and shout "*ciao!*" (*good-bye!*) to the rest. This philosophy has proved incredibly valuable on occasions I have suspected or I have been told I may have a serious health issue that needed further investigation. On those occasions, diagnostic blood tests or biopsies were taken.

In the week between undergoing diagnostic tests and learning the results, I fought emotional entrapment by stepping outside of how I felt about the potential diagnosis and analyzing it from an outsider's view—a rather surreal examination. The key was to move from the inner emotional realm and examine the situation from an external outlook. The external view allowed me to take an objective account, set aside pieces over which I had no control and more clearly identify pieces I could effect.

As an example, when I awaited the result of a biopsy to rule out cancer, I focused on identifying the choices I had in both the best and worst scenarios. More often than not, diagnostic tests confirmed no cancer or illness. I reminded myself that statistics were on the positive side. *You cannot control the outcome of the test at this point so let go of trying to control the outcome.* I diverted my thoughts from hopelessness, telling myself that if the test came back positive for cancer I still had the power to choose treatment. And if I chose aggressive treatment I could choose rearranging my life schedule to refocus energies on my healing and let go of the small activities that usurped my daily time. In other words, I had control over many items no matter what the diagnosis.

Release all the worrisome thoughts before you hear from the doctor. "Coraggio."

If I felt it would be helpful to talk about the situation during limbo week I confided in one person. I reassured her there was no need to worry while waiting for test results and I felt assured. There was no need to spread worry to anyone before confirmation. All I needed from her now was to be able to talk through my plan and to pray with her. Prayer for me built a fortress of hope and despair dissolved in a wisp.

I had witnessed how the opposite approach had a detrimental impact on a person and everyone in her wake. A co-worker received a call from her doctor's office while at the workplace recommending she have a follow-up mammogram sometime in the next couple of weeks. They kindly reassured her that often mammogram tests have a high rate of false positives. Before she hung up the phone the coworker fell apart, uncontrollably sobbing at her workstation. None of the other office staff could console her, despite giving her hugs and uttering soothing comments. Although it was the middle of the work day a friend had to come to our office, pick her up and drive her home because she was too upset to drive. The coworker then called the doctor's office several times that day and with such inconsolable hysteria that the doctor's staff pulled strings to arrange a mammogram the following day. The second mammogram showed no breast tissue abnormalities; the first mammogram had been flawed.

I tell this story not to be critical of the coworker, but rather to point out that *you* are in control of your mindset and behavior that you will adopt for any situation. Think about the variety of attitudes available to espouse; then think about wearing that attitude. How does the attitude make you feel about yourself? How does the attitude help you to manage or cope with your situation? Does the attitude you have chosen help you feel empowered and help you retain the energy you need to deal with the situation, or does the attitude you have chosen overwhelm you so that you feel powerless, stressed and drained?

Now envision the impact the attitude you have chosen will have on the individuals around you. Is your attitude spinning off and spreading negative stress to those around you, or is your attitude assisting others to form a cohesive front of support for you? In the coworker's case, she disrupted an entire business office, and emotionally upset herself, her family and her friends. The friend who picked up the coworker in the middle of the day to drive her home lost a half day of work and was unexpectedly not available to support the staff at a separate workplace. The coworker herself lost a day and a half of work for nothing she could change at the time she got the call suggesting a follow-up mammogram.

Moral of the story: If you cannot control the outcome, let go of any emotion or efforts that do not bring peace to you and those around you.

Setting aside emotions in health situations, especially situations involving life or death, may seem callously unrealistic. At first I had to consciously shift into a business-like mode. Now that I am more aware and practiced, this conscious shift technique occurs more easily. I switch from an emotional framework approach to health, to a business approach. In this business model I view myself as a sophisticated businesswoman. I protect my business by making sure I stay on the cutting edge of advances in my field, by having adequate assets, by not taking foolish risks, and by faithfully carrying liability insurance.

To apply the business analogy to my health, I am constantly seeking information on healthy living and in treatment advances for my illnesses. I eat well, exercise, get adequate sleep, carry health insurance and seek a doctor when necessary. I feel secure in the business I have built. My business is dependent on me approaching any profit or loss situation with a calm, non-emotional approach. I learn all the facts and analyze all the options. Weighing all pros and cons I make a measured and practical decision that is best for my business.

Accordingly, when a health challenge arises, I flip into the business analogy and turn off the emotions. I learn all I can from the doctor, the nurse, the health insurance company and my own research. I calmly and deliberately analyze all the facts and options with my health professionals and support system.

People have asked me, "How can you deal with this without being upset or emotional?" That is exactly the point. Would I make important decisions critical to my business in an emotional manner? If I did, not only would the chances of me making a poor choice be likely, I would be wasting a tremendous amount of energy needed to run other aspects of the business, not to mention cause turmoil to my staff. To me, it makes better sense when dealing with my health, which is paramount to any business deal, that I would also approach it in a calm, measured and deliberate manner?

With courage it is possible to:

- Remove yourself from the emotional realm of a health crisis in order to clearly view areas you can positively impact.

- Remove yourself from the emotional realm of a health crisis to foster inner tranquility.

- Say "ciao" to and let go of worry about matters over which you have no control and actions that cannot positively change an outcome.

CHAPTER 27

Denial as a Means of Control

DENIAL IS A MEANS OF CONTROL. I OFTEN FORGET I AM A PERSON LIVING with two chronic, serious illnesses, have two artificial knees, screws and plates in my ankles, wires in my chest, and crater scars from two occurrences of basal cell cancer. A healthy dose of denial always helped my "can do" attitude.

Not dwelling on my health situation may be denying it to a certain degree, but when presented with a potential adventure the denial helps me to jump at the thought of "I can!" instead of "Oh no. I can't." I recognize that by employing denial I may end up walking too far or overexerting myself. As a result of the overexertion my feet, ankles, knees and hips may hurt more than usual for a couple of days or my leg muscles may be fatigued for a stretch.

For me, experiencing the adventure was a good trade-off. I do try to be judicious with the denial however and not enter a situation which may harm my joints or exacerbate either disease. I place a big neon-flashing warning sign over the pop-psychology talk of "embracing" your illness.

Embrace your life. Embrace your loved ones. Embrace your faith. Embrace what is good around you. But be cautious if the pop-psychologists urge you to embrace the negative aspects of your disease. Do not lie down and accept every bad aspect of an illness you hear or read about. Fight it and beat it. Do not accept symptoms that have <u>not</u> occurred. Do not embrace or surrender to the disease! *Coraggio* is the battle cry!

It takes courage to:

- Say "I can!" instead of "I can't."
- Not passively accept a non-manifested symptom merely because you read about it.
- Discern the difference between healthy denial and denial which could lead to harm.

CHAPTER 28

Caution Against Controlling Others as a Means of Control

I NEED TO EXPRESS CAUTIONARY LIMITS AS I ENCOURAGE TO CONTROL WHAT you can. My desire to express caution stems from an experience for which, more than twenty years later, I feel ashamed. Controlling other people is also a means of control. Be careful not to manipulate relationships in the guise of taking charge of your own life. Controlling your own actions and choices is not the same as controlling other people's actions or choices.

When I was 23 years old, similar to most of my peers, I thought I was fully emotionally mature. I thought I had relationships figured out. I thought I was enlightened on issues of compassion and on the give-and-take philosophy. Boy, did I need illumination.

I spent half of my 23rd and all of my 24th year in a wheelchair. Much of it I spent in bed, joints locked in pain and almost entirely reliant on my mother and grandmother for food, toileting and bathing. My mother and I believed that I could be cured using natural means to rebuild cartilage that had been eaten away between my knees and other joints using fresh produce to ensure that I was taking in live vitamins, enzymes and minerals that could be used as building locks for physiological restoration.

Each morning my mother would arise at 5:00 a.m. and pray for half an hour. In that dim, early hour she would then take the many organic carrots my grandmother had scrubbed the night before and force them through our high-tech juicer until about 12 ounces of healing juice was produced. She would then head to my bedroom, orange-frothed glass in hand, open my window shades, whisper a sweet greeting, and kneel at the side of my bed, careful not to spill the vital contents in the tall, amber-pearled, ribbed glass. My elbows were so painfully locked in a flexed position, especially in the morning, that my mother would gently lift my head, hold the glass to my lips and wait patiently for me to ingest the thick, sweet, orange-colored, carrot liquid. On one particular morning I took an unexpectedly large gulp of frigid carrot juice and shrieked in protest. With unkind tone I complained that the juice was too cold to drink so quickly.

Looking back a few years later, and after my mother had died, I saw the scenario from a different viewpoint. Yes, the juice was cold because the carrots had been refrigerated through the night. The previous night innumerable carrots had been dutifully scrubbed by a selfless grandmother so that it would be less-time consuming for a selfless mother who in the pre-dawn, pre-work hours sought to prepare a health-yielding drink for her daughter. My mother had to be exhausted from this early morning routine, but she never complained. She must have been concerned that she had to get ready for work, but she never exhibited impatience. When she had tipped the liquid carrot-filled glass at my lips and the big cold gulp had unintentionally resulted, I had sputtered and objected. I didn't want cold carrot juice and I wanted it in smaller gulps!

Looking back at the incident through the wiser eyes I realized that part of my behavior had stemmed from wanting control. I did not have control over my health or activities of daily living. So in a pathetic grasp for control, I tried to control my mother by blaming her for a big, cold gulp.

I am profoundly sad as I reflect on my behavior. The sadness is deepened as I realize that because her death occurred soon after the incident, I had not recognized my control issues and never had an opportunity to apologize to her. I never had and never will be able to embrace her in thanksgiving for all she did those early mornings. But I can write about the detriment in trying to control others as a means of feeling more control for yourself.

The caregiver-patient relationship is complicated, especially if the caregiver or patient is a family member or significant other. I know how difficult it can be to feel dependent and have to rely on others. I know the conundrum of being grateful for assistance while simultaneously being unhappy because the service is not up to your standard or preference.

I am not sure I have the optimal answer to the challenge, so for now I try to take an honest look at my thoughts, motivations, words and actions. I put myself on guard for any behavior that hints of trying to unreasonably control another person's choice or action. In place of criticism I focus on appreciating the caregiver or friend for the assistance. In other words, I banish the critical thoughts and release frustrated feelings about the task not being performed the way I prefer.

> *Why did she fold my laundry that way? That is not how laundry is folded. What took her so long, anyway? I was without clean socks for two days.*

> *I can't believe he bought me green apples instead of red apples. He knows I don't like green apples.*

Instead I express gratitude: *I am so thankful that she did all my laundry. Now I have clean clothing and bedding.*

And I take responsibility for my part in any conflict and acknowledge the effort put forth from a heart desirous of helping me: *Thank you for shopping so I have fresh, healthy produce to eat. I am sorry I only wrote "apples" on the shopping list and caused confusion for you as you stood amid 12 varieties of apples trying to figure out which apples would please me the most.*

When I am feeling as if I am losing control over my health or my life, bossing someone around is not going to resolve the reason behind my feeling of loss or helplessness. Taking a seat on my high horse of superiority is only going to add feelings of dissatisfaction to my feelings of helplessness. More productive for me and for those who care for me, is to grab courage, and with it a piece of humble pie. With courage, humility and gratitude I can try to do as much as I can for myself and feel appreciation for the help I receive from others.

With courage it is possible to:

- Recognize that in every circumstance your choice of attitude and whether to express gratitude will have an impact on the people around you.

- Recognize that you may be trying to control others in order to feel you are in control of your own life.

- Recognize that the demanding, ungrateful behavior of the person for whom you are providing care may be rooted in their feelings of loss of independence and control.

- Say "thank you" or "I appreciate you" even if you would have preferred the task performed in another manner or sooner.

- Seek the support of others when you feel helpless instead of pushing them away with demanding behavior.

- Transform feelings of frustration into expressions of gratitude.

- Accept help from others with grace and humility.

CHAPTER 29
Taking Charge of Grief

GRANDFATHER (NONNO) GIGLIOTTI PASSED AWAY IN FALL OF 1978. NONNA was only 66 years old. Grandpa had been Nonna's life partner for almost 50 years. He was a loud, vibrant, social man. He loved life, people, food and music, and he loved his grandchildren more than anything else in the world.

Grandpa's larger-than-life personality left delightful and vivid images in my mind. I recall those images now, captured and memorialized from a young girl's perspective. Standing in his small living room; the audience of four grandchildren seated in a row on the couch facing him with anticipatory glee as he loudly, jovially, bellowed a rendition of the Julius La Rosa classic song, "*Eh Compari!*"

Eh compari, ci vo sunari. Chi si sona? U friscalettu.
E comu si sona u friscalettu?
U friscalette, tipiti tipiti tam.

(Hey, buddy! Let's make some music.
What'll I play?
The piccolo.)

I was uncertain what the Italian words meant but I guessed from the actions he made as he held his finger-flickering hands to the side of his animated face that he was imitating playing the *friscalettu* (piccolo). As the subject of the frivolous but catchy ditty moved from one musical instrument to the next, so did Grandpa's animations for the *saxofona, mandolinu, violinu, trumbetta,* and *trombona,* all the while Grandpa singing loudly in Italian, eyes fixed on us, his lips, cheeks and eyebrows dramatically accentuating his melodic tale for his grandkids. Paintings rattled against the wall, photo frames shivered on their surfaces as Grandpa attempted to rapidly shift his massive body weight from one foot to another in *tarantella* hopping fashion, his adoring miniature fans giggling and laughing until doubled over in their seated row. Oh Lord, we loved Grandpa. Oh Lord, he made us laugh.

Each Sunday Grandpa prominently sat at the head of his kitchen table, all four of us grandchildren mesmerized as he told noisy stories, accompanied by fist pounding, extravagant impersonations, and thunderous laughter. We barely noticed Nonna, quietly cooking or cleaning dishes behind us. Outside of family and a few neighbors, Nonna's social circle consisted of the people who Grandpa invited for a slain wildlife dinner or to sample from his basement wine cellar while Nonna silently prepared food or dutifully cleaned the remnants of entertaining.

Nonna and her two sisters never learned to drive. All three Rizzo daughters married Italian-born men with Old Country ideas of what was expected of women; driving was not one of the expectations. Nonna did not handle the household finances either nor had she her own source of income since she stopped working when she give birth to her second child 30 years prior.

Our family feared without Grandpa, Nonna would wither and die, as Nonna's life revolved around a vivacious man who was no longer physically present. Grieving the loss of one held dear is so vast, a tiny, meek, widow like Nonna could be swallowed into its unrelenting cold darkness. We could not imagine a way for her to conquer home ownership, develop her own identity, and survive.

But we should never have underestimated Nonna *"testadura"* Gigliotti. Soon after Grandpa died, Nonna prodded Uncle Matt, her sister Angelina's husband, to drive her to the closest bank. She courageously opened her own checking account and had someone teach her how to manage the checkbook, then asked us grandchildren to review the checkbook periodically to ensure she was doing okay. She solicited information about the city taxes on her home and how to pay them. She set up her own system of putting modest amounts of money from her Social Security check into a new savings account so she could pay the annual taxes. And at almost 70 years of age she got her first credit card!

With the long, isolating Michigan winter approaching we feared Nonna would slide into depression alone in her small home without Grandpa and his beloved backyard garden that consumed so much of their time from spring until fall. But there was no depression for Nonna. She found ways to occupy her mind and hands so that depression never had a chance. She left Grandpa's bed, chest and dresser in his bedroom and reconfigured a corner to be the sewing space she always wanted. She took old cardboard boxes and covered them with contact paper. Into the neatly covered boxes Nonna organized and stored all her sewing material and notions. She spent the rest of the winter planning the backyard garden.

While Grandpa was alive, every inch of their backyard garden was vegetables, fruit and flowers. Even the concrete slab patio on which we dined and gathered in the summer was thickly covered overhead with dense, fruit-swollen grape vines. It was daunting to believe that Nonna alone could maintain Grandpa's garden. But she was determined to make the garden and our Sunday gatherings Grandpa's legacy. She arrived at solutions by beginning with smaller pieces she knew she could handle. She searched through seed catalogs, staring out the kitchen window and contemplating the garden, now covered with snow, occasional patches of dead grass and brown fallen leaves. She let go of the desire for the vegetables that were the most burdensome to grow and instead bought low maintenance flowers that she had dreamed would fill her surroundings and her life with beauty. She could order the catalog seeds and bulbs and pay with her own check or credit card. All this she did by believing there was a solution and taking control.

As many Europeans have known, life is full of adversity and never ending change. Instead of complaining about it, she adapted and moved on. It took her the entire winter, but Nonna had searched for and found ways to take charge of her grief and her life. Instead of giving up on hope, she focused on all the things she could do before spring's arrival. As long as she was alive the idea of a garden was alive.

Nonna's positive focus led to the creation of a lush and prosperous garden. She had accomplished Grandpa's legacy of sweet-smelling, soothing, nourishing, green vegetation. And she would still have her son and grandchildren for Sunday dinner, often feeding us with the incredible harvest from her garden.

What I would give for a bowl of Nonna's Italian pole beans the vines of which Nonna had affectionately tied to six feet high poles with strips of soft cloth she had torn from old t-shirts or bed sheets. Under her loving care the one-inch wide green bean would merrily grow to eight inches in length. Fresh-picked and par-boiled, Nonna mixed the pot of tender beans with cloves she had pulled from the garlic patch by the chain-link fence that bordered the east side of her yard. Most people have no idea garlic fresh pulled from the ground is translucent, and upon slicing, beads and oozes the intense garlic essence for which it is beloved around the world. With beans still steaming from its hot bath, basil picked only moments before from densely leaved bushes were mixed with the beans and garlic. Traditionally boiled potatoes were added, but at times the magical medley was served unadulterated by potato. *Mmmm.* Pungent garlic and crisp basil essence fills the nostrils one second before the flavor bursts.

Nonna not only learned how to become independent after Grandpa's death, but in the process her harvests were as much a delight to the palate as they were a comfort for the soul.

I can still picture myself standing in the narrow space between two tall rows of Nonna's Italian pole beans. The vines have grown above my height so that I am enveloped in the dense, bright green, heart-shaped leaves. I feel the warmth of the sun penetrating the leaves, contributing to the green hue. I hear the buzz of flies and bees, yet in the background plays the memory of Grandpa's contented whistle of a peppy Italian cantata. I smell the sun-warmed, green vegetation and moist soil.

In this vibrant space surrounded by abundant life I am reminded of how Nonna took charge of her grief and kept Grandpa's spirit alive and I am reminded that I, too, can take charge in any challenge and turn it into a positive.

A few yards away from the imagined row of Italian pole beans is the spot where Nonna stood to cast her *il malocchio* curse and set the course for taking charge of the rain run-off flood in her life. And with her actions came for me *Lezione Due* (Lesson Two): a lesson on mustering courage to take charge of the aspects of life I can control.

You, too, have control over how you live your life, but it takes courage.

"Coraggio, Leeza."

In challenging situations I try to step back, look at the bigger picture, and find an aspect that I can manage. It might be as minuscule a change as to tell myself to let go: "fo-getta 'bout it". I may not be able to change the situation, but I guarantee I will find a part of it I can.

With courage it is possible to:

- Transform grief into a loved one's legacy.
- Thwart depression by finding purpose in your life and working daily to fulfill that purpose.

Lezione Tre: Amore
(Lesson Three: Love)

The Courage to Love Yourself
When You Feel Unlovable;
The Courage to Love
Another Despite Being Hurt;
The Courage to Feel Love
Again After the Loss of
One You Love

Chapter 30
The Big Italian Family Fight

THERE WAS WAILING AND THERE WAS FLAILING. THERE WAS SOME CURSING in English and a whole lot of invoking the Blessed Virgin Mary in Italian.

"*O Madonna Mia … O Madonna M-eeee-a!*" was the repeated pathetic cry from Nonna that tore through her son and her grandchildren.

Our Italian-American family favors the passive-aggressive method of communication and issue resolution. Any Italian-American knows exactly what I am talking about. On rare occasions there was the "Big Italian Family Fight" and this family fight was the worst ever.

Nonna was born in Southern Italy, which was notorious for the genetic personality trait of "*testadura*" (hard-head). At 88 years old at the time, she had just been released from another cardiac unit hospital stay. Once again her doctors, nurses and social workers had said it was unsafe for her to live in her home by herself. We had known for almost two years that her deteriorating health required a move, but there was no such convincing hard-headed Nonna Gigliotti. Nothing could make her move from the small, blue-collar home that she and Grandpa Francesco had labored, scrimped and saved most of their adult lives to buy, and with all of the pride of the Calabrese Italian, their home was their own.

My sister, Laura, and I, the two granddaughters, were exhausted from administering most of the care to Nonna. Tired of the decades-long cycle of passive-aggressive behavior, we decided to commence a family meeting. My father Pasquale, Nonna's only living child, my two brothers, sister, and I assembled in Nonna's tiny living room. *La Famiglia* (the family) was seated on her floral couch, her pink velour easy chairs and the taupe-carpeted floor facing Nonna. The photo of Father Solanus on the wall behind her and the painting of Pope John Paul II to her right, hung as if poised to guard her.

The heavy air of dread thickened with tension. The meeting did not achieve the peaceful resolution Laura and I had envisioned. Instead, there was Nonna, fresh from a hospital stay for her failing heart, throwing herself up and down from her pink velour recliner, arms flinging, voice at a strained pitch never heard before. "If yous make me move I … I'll call the papers and tell them what yous are doing to me …" Nonna knew how to thrust the guilt knife into my heart.

My brother, Peter, the oldest Italian grandson, was akin to God. Visibly shaken by Nonna's emotional reaction, he turned to Laura and me. "You are not going to do anything to upset

MY grandmother!" His pointed finger was inches from my sister's face but his threat was aimed at both of us.

HIS grandmother? I was fuming.

What an outrageous statement from him who had performed relatively little of the hands-on help for HIS grandmother in recent years!

My father, to whom the caregiver responsibility should have fallen as Nonna's only living child, sat speechless through the entire fight, thoroughly unprepared for the unexpectedly dramatic conflict. *Dad, why can't you take charge?!* His stunned inaction added to my shocked disbelief at how quickly the situation was turning disastrous.

But the worst was yet to come. The grandmother I adored executed the dreaded silent treatment. The meeting was over; the flames of the fiery fight snuffed by Nonna's chilling impenetrable snub.

It was not safe for Nonna to live alone in her home. Pent up frustrations from all family members had exploded and been aired, but the issue of Nonna's safety continued.

I was her best friend. I knew the way her mind worked. I knew what she was thinking.

"Lisa betrayed me. She was the person I trusted the most, yet she betrayed me. She is supposed to take care of me in my old age and instead she wants to move me to a nursing home. I will show her. I will take care of myself in my own home without her help. I will never talk to her again!"

"Darn the *testadura!*"

My heart was breaking. I was shaken by how distressed the usually gentle, frail Nonna had become. I was stinging from the Nonna-protecting bully gesture of my older brother toward my sister and me. I was disappointed that my father had not taken a leadership role, and as a consequence left my sister and me as the bad guys. I felt guilty for spearheading an effort that had gone terribly wrong and created the platform for explosive emotions and hurt feelings. Adrenalin-laden blood expanded the vessels at my neck with forcible throbs and pounded in my ears. My face felt flushed, my palms sweaty and cold.

As the trembling subsided I felt as if I would be sick to my stomach. I had internalized and ruminated on all the negative feelings spinning from the Big Italian Family Fight. I was unable to process my feelings with my sister because in her woundedness she would not talk to anyone, especially me, who had drafted her into the idea of a family meeting. I could not explain to Nonna that my plan was based on compassionate concern for her safety and health.

Nonna would not utter a word to me.

"*Pieta, Nonna. Pieta.*" (Have mercy, Nonna. Mercy.)

"No!" the message of her cold silence.

My brothers and father were to be avoided out of fear of me causing further family turmoil.

Without venting any of the raw emotion, I went to bed with an awful mix of sadness, frustration and anger stewing inside. "*O Dio, aiutarci!*" (O God, help us)

I woke up the next day in the tranquil fortress of my own home. Before I even opened my eyes *pain* signals began to enter my brain, reporting from several body parts, violently ricocheting back to the body part resulting in the sensation of being brutally smashed with a hammer. My head pressed tightly into the pillow, bracing against the pain. I tried to switch my focus from thinking of the pain before it became overwhelming, but with horror I realized I could not open my hands or unbend my elbow. I forced against searing flames to raise my arm, bend my elbow and twist my wrist so I could view my hand. Each motion brought screeching protest from the joint involved. I was shocked to see the visible increase of redness and swelling in my hands, wrists and elbows. I used the momentum from my torso to swing my legs to the side of the bed and sit at the edge. Gingerly I stepped down on my feet and tried to stand. My feet and ankles felt as if I had stepped on the sharp end of four inch nails, two piercing entirely through the foot and two plunging deep into the center of the ankle joint. It was impossible to step down. I could not walk!

If ever I held skepticism about a mind-body connection it vanished that morning. To my knowledge I had not inflicted any physical trauma or exertion to my hands and feet to merit such a drastic inflammatory response. I had taken all medications according to doctors' orders. I had not eaten salty food that might have caused joint swelling. The only variance to my daily routine was the prior day's violent emotional assault. I had allowed myself to fully absorb feelings of hurt, frustration, guilt and injustice. Then I allowed the toxic brew of tormenting emotions to fester all night. In effect, I had allowed the Big Italian Family Fight to throw a knock-out punch.

With courage you can:
- Recognize that thoughts and feelings may effect physical health.
- Learn not to dwell on negative thoughts and feelings.

CHAPTER 31

Self-Love

I BELIEVED MYSELF TO BE "MISS POSITIVE." I BELIEVED THAT THROUGH CONSTANT self-examination and attempts to improve my inner-self I had cleaned out a lot of negative emotions and had achieved a center of peace and equanimity. I had dealt with tough challenges and believed that I could deal with whatever came my way. Or so I thought.

Upon waking in the morning, my eyes would open, and I would reprimand myself. *Why did you go to bed so late? Now you are going to be tired all day!*

After hobbling into the bathroom, I would turn sideways and smooth my pajama top to examine my profile in the mirror. *Why did you eat so much food yesterday? Now your waistline is bulging!*

You are going to look fat in anything you wear today and it is your own fault! Combine the bulging belly with the dark circles under your eyes and you will win the beauty prize for the day!

This self-critical routine would be played out repeatedly through the years until one morning I realized that the first messages I said to myself were negative and damaging. I would never have allowed a friend or an enemy to address me in such a negative manner nor would I have held true the words they spoke. Why then did I allow myself to talk to me so cruelly?

The concept of self-love is important to me. There are many books on healing which focus on a body-mind or metaphysical approach to healing one's self. These theorists point out that the source of many chronic diseases is the body attacking itself. They propose that the root of the disease can be determined by examining the inner self to discover why the body might be attacking itself. For example, not liking yourself on an emotional level sends the same self-dislike message on the body's cellular level; eventually your own cells turn against each other. In this proposition the cure is achieved by removing the bad self-thoughts so that the body's cells will in turn fall into self-allegiance.

I have a ferocious battle occurring within my body in that it is being attacked by my own cells. That in essence is what the term autoimmune means. To use the old Greek Trojan horse analogy, the horse is met with glee, perceived by the body as a needed part of the immune response. But the warriors within, when released, slaughter the good. Because I have two autoimmune diseases, both of which are severe, I have given this metaphysical theory a lot of consideration. I was raised Italian-Catholic and inherited the double dose of shame and guilt that accompanies the cultural-religious combination. My modus operandi is *Mea Culpa*. (I am guilty and it's my fault). No one can ever be more critical of me than me.

Both rheumatoid arthritis and myasthenia gravis are autoimmune diseases. Another way of thinking of "autoimmune" is

"self-immune." In very simple terms, the destruction of rheumatoid arthritis comes from the cells of my body that are supposed
to defend against infection invaders. Instead, the immune cells
attack the healthy cells of all my joints. Similarly in myasthenia
gravis, a messenger is sent by the nerve to lock into a specific
niche on the muscle and as a result activate the muscle into motion. Instead, my body makes an imposter messenger that stuffs
itself into the cubby-hole, therefore blocking the true messenger
from entering and enabling the muscle to move.

You may be saying, the mind-body connection is a bunch
of new age hooey. That is okay and I hope there is some other
morsel in this book that helps you. It does have logic enough to
earn at least some merit. And if you are a person with a chronic
and potentially debilitating or deadly disease, you will try just
about anything to promote healing. The recipe for cure is harm-
less. While the body-mind books suggest I stand in front of the
mirror and repeat, "I Love You, Lisa", for me it was a big enough
step just to recognize all the negative self-talk that was going on.
Now if I start with critical self-talk, I gently bring the negative
thoughts to a stop and fill the negative thought spot with something positive such as, "I am so grateful I can stand on both feet
today. Thank you feet!" Or "I am excited I will spend time with a
good friend today!"

Sometimes it is difficult to love yourself because of the ignorance of a stranger or the insecurity of a friend. There are many
people who have not had a lot of exposure to people with disabilities and have a perception that if you are in a wheelchair
because your legs do not work it also means that your brain does
not work.

During the three-year stint a wheelchair was my only means
of mobility, I decided to fly from Los Angeles to Detroit to visit
family. My mother drove me to LAX International Airport and
navigated its extensive distance through harried throngs to my
departure gate. My mother, with her long-legged strides, answered

the call for wheelchair assistance pre-boarding by wheeling me to the jet way.

Upon reaching the ticket-taking podium the airline worker ignored me, looked at my mother instead and asked, "Can she walk to the bathroom by herself?"

It was as if the fact that my legs did not work automatically meant that my brain could not possibly work.

"I'm not sure; why don't you ask her?" was my mother's instant response, never releasing the ignorant worker's glance.

My humiliation turned to uncharitable thoughts. *There is a good possibility I have more years of education and a greater intelligence quota than you. I may not be able to walk but I can answer just fine!*

While critical and hurtful thoughts may come from ignorant or impolite strangers, comments from friends can carry a more burning sting. Friends have declined to split an order of food, apologizing for their fear of contracting rheumatoid arthritis. Before visiting their homes, siblings of friends have inquired whether I might carry rheumatoid arthritis to their children. Rheumatoid arthritis is not contagious and cannot be transmitted from one human to another. Yet it was easy to personalize the fear and comments into shameful hurt.

I mention the stories of negative impact to illustrate the importance of possessing an impenetrable barrier of self-love. It is difficult to love yourself when your body does not match "beautiful" as society has painted beauty. It is difficult to feel self-worth if you have gone from an active lifestyle or successful career to a status that appears somehow not as successful or not as independent. A strong love for self is critical.

Without a fortress of self-love the negative messages society sends can stealthily creep in and slowly erode self-worth or can commit a blistering attack on belief in your good. My experience as a person with severe disabilities living in Michigan during the pro-assisted suicide movement of the 1990s taught me that often people with disabilities presume their life is not worthy because society or a person tells them they are burden or a scourge. The majority of women Jack Kevorkian assisted to die did not have terminal illnesses; background facts actually showed most of them had depression. Many of the women had left stories of how their husbands, boyfriends or families had told them they were unworthy or a burden.

I knew I needed to work through the remnants of the beliefs about myself I had collected throughout my life and to throw out those that no longer fit or those that do not serve to solidify my belief that I have worth.

It took a lot of courage to go through that emotional closet, to hold out each remnant before me for an honest inspection. But I knew that a solid foundation in self-worth was essential to me liking and loving myself. I must be ever vigilant to resist the temptation to consider critical self-thought and negative self-talk. And for me, temptation is more difficult to fight when I am fatigued or in pain. But the fight to believe in and feel the love I have for me is worth it now that I am aware of my own mind-body connection and what it means for my health.

With courage you can:

- Be vigilant to detect and resist critical self-thought and negative self-talk.

- Replace critical self-thought and negative self-talk with love-talk.

- Discover the mind-body connections that may be negatively affecting your health.

- Discover the mind-body connections that may be positively affecting your health.

CHAPTER 32

The Importance of Positive Attitude in Achieving Self=Love, Less Pain and Life Gusto

POSITIVE ATTITUDE HELPED ME TO SURVIVE THE MONTHS I WAS BEDRIDDEN. The statement seems simple, even trite. But the meaning behind "positive attitude helped me to survive" in this context is interconnected with many aspects of my life. Positive attitude affects how I feel about myself, how I see myself in relation to the universe, how others perceive me, and the disposition of my interactions with others.

As I experienced after the Big Italian Family Fight, physical tissues erupted in an inflamed response to my emotional upheaval. My perception of being stuck in a situation that was exasperating, had no good solution, and in which I had been "bad" by fanning flames of family frustration, resulted in a negative attitude about my world and about myself. WHAM! My body hurt and my feelings of frustration multiplied.

During my early twenties when fierce arthritis caused me to be bedridden and mobile only by wheelchair, positive attitude brought me hope that I would soon be healthy enough to join my classmates in medical school. Positive attitude fostered strive to do everything possible to heal. The alternative would have been to feel sorry for myself and deteriorate physically as I deteriorated emotionally into depression. I believe having a positive attitude brought more willingness on the part of friends and family to interact with me than if I had been whiny, weepy or grumpy. If I held a positive attitude about myself and my situation, I was more likely to be gracious, kind and grateful toward my caregivers.

But how could I awake with a positive attitude after spending the long, dark hours of night wrestling with tortuous pain? How could I spend my day maintaining a positive attitude when I was not sitting in the medical school classroom with other students my age? How could I derive one moment of positive attitude while locked in an arthritic-balled position in my bed? Let me tell you, it took *coraggio*. A lot of courage.

On many mornings I had to work for the positive attitude. Rather than think of it as work, I thought of it as the "Oh Happy Day" game. But there were mornings I had to force my mind into the happy day mode.

It was by my mother's example that I learned the rules to the little game of achieving daily positive attitude. Each day she would rise at 5:30 a.m. She would spend the next half hour in prayer and meditation. By the time she reached my bedroom she was revved with cheer and gleaming with a smile.

"Good morning, Sunshine!" *Phalooop!* Up went the noisy bedroom window blinds, flooding my room with the dawning California sunshine.

Okay. I was awake, but the morning joint pain seemed sharper than what I had endured throughout the night. *Oh God.* I could not even unbend my elbows from the pain-locked position of forearms crossed over my belly.

With springing steps my mother turned from the window and reached the side of my bed. With perfect ballet-grace she landed gently at my bedside, perched on folded knees. I knew she did not like to see my elbows locked at the 90-degree angle, fearing the physical therapist's heed that without extension of the muscles, joint contractures could set in.

"It's a gorgeous day! The sun is bright and the sky is really blue today."

Okay. Her visual brought my mind to a land of glowing sunshine and blue skies.

"Let's try to unbend your elbows, Sweet Pea, so they do not get frozen in a bent position. C'mon, let's move them now so that I can help you sit up."

"*Arrrrrrrrgh!*" the sharp, stabbing pain was unbearable as the elbow ground to an open position as she moved each arm off my belly. I yelped and clenched my jaw. *Oohhhh.* The jaw cracked in painful echo.

"I cannot wait to get you up and bring you to the balcony so you can see the hummingbird that is feeding off the flowers on the hanging fuchsia plant. It is amazing to see it up close while it flits about."

Okay. Her visual brought me to the curiosity center of my mind. What color was the bird? Would I see the blur of its fast-flickering wings? Was its beak nature's evolution of a perfect nectar extractor? *Wow.* My mother had stolen me from the pain center of my mind and I did not even know it.

She now placed her arm around my shoulder and back to help me slowly lift my torso into a partly raised position. She held the glass to my lips so I could drink the fresh carrot juice she had prepared. She came back after I used the bedside commode, helped me swing into my wheelchair and wheeled me out onto the balcony. I stared up at the bright, dark pink fuchsia flowers. The morning sun enhanced the rich color and velvety softness of the fuchsia's petals. Within two minutes a hummingbird appeared, its wings flapping so furiously it looked akin to a bee. It truly did have a long, spiked nose used to busily enter the center of each flower to gather sweet sustenance. A joy sprung forth from the center of my chest and spread up toward my throat. In that moment happiness permeated my being. I was witness to a melding of nature's most spectacular: sun, sky, flower, hummingbird. "*La Dolce Vita*" (The sweet life). Life was good!

My mother's smile glistened and in my memory it is as if her radiating smile was larger than life. Her shoulders were raised toward her ears in delight as if a child experiencing a first moment of excitement. Then I listened to her "favorite things" phrases I heard her gush hundreds of times: "Everyday I am grateful for living in California. I can go to the ocean or go to the mountains all in the same day! I am so fortunate to live in this climate. All the sunshine! It is cool in the mornings, warm during the day, and then cool again in the evening. Just perfect!"

Her mantra of gratitude perpetuated throughout the day. While driving me home at night she would slow the car to a stop at the side of a road lined by dark silhouettes of tall, thin trees. She reached across me to roll down the manual window because my pain-wracked elbows were no longer capable. "Close your eyes and take a deep breath. Do you smell that? It is from the eucalyptus trees on this road. Only in Southern California! We are so fortunate!"

When we pulled into the driveway of the home she and my Hungarian grandmother shared, she sped around the back of the car, opened my door, and before helping me out would say, "Close your eyes and take a deep breath. Do you smell that? It is from the wild rosemary bushes growing all around the house. Isn't it wonderful? Aren't we blessed to be surrounded by rosemary?"

Sometimes when I pointed out that she had missed the turn-off to their house she would respond, "You will see." And with a wide grin she would stare at the treacherously winding road as it continued to cut and curl through the Malibu canyon. At the point when I thought her old small car could no longer endure the steep pull she would swing onto an almost hidden turnoff. From the perch she would show me the miles and miles of rolling hills below us, viewed from every bit of a 360-degree horizon. The Southern California brush dotting the hillsides were dyed purple from the setting sun, peach hue emanating up to meet what was left of the perpetual blue sky.

"To the left, just over that farthest hill, is the Pacific Ocean. Look down, over to the right. That is where they film the *M.A.S.H.* television show. Can you believe the colors of the land-scape? Can't you just feel the majesty? Thank you, God that we are able to be present and partake of this view". And then, prompted by purple hues and mounded emblems of majesty, she would be off ... singing *America the Beautiful*, " ... *for purple mountain majesty* ... " with all the joy in her heart as loud as her lungs could produce. To this day I can hear her proud pure tones echoing through the canyon pass as it bounced from one hillside to another. It was like living with Julie Andrews (Maria Von Trapp from the *Sound of Music*).

My mother was tall, slender, blonde and blue-eyed like Julie Andrews, and she had a perky and angelic-voice like Julie Andrews, too. Starting each day with my mother was right out of a scene from *The Sound of Music* scene where Maria, attempting to abate the Von Trapp children's fear of a thunderstorm by having them focus on positive thoughts, clutches her bedroom window drapery and sings "My Favorite Things."

Just as Maria had provided the Von Trapp children the tools to think of favorite things so they would not "feel so bad," so had my mother provided me the tools to garner positive thoughts. I had been filled with wonder at watching the hummingbird and fuchsia. I had felt the splendor and majesty of the purple, rolling mountains. I felt blessed to smell eucalyptus and rosemary from where I was sitting or to know I lived where the sun shone most days on aqua ocean, purple mountains and green valleys. I had observed my mother derive such joy, satisfaction, and gratitude for even common things that pass by most people each day. She had an ongoing list of all the things for which she was grateful, and as she went through an accounting of her list of treasures, her joy and positive attitude swelled. You want to talk about "power tools"? Knowing how to formulate and use the "Oh, Happy Day" list was one of the most powerful tools my mother could have ever gifted to me.

During the bedridden months I called on those tools. At times I had to *force* myself into completing the "Oh, Happy Day" game. The positive list did not appear in my mind or heart when I awoke, wracked in pain, struggling against my feelings of disappointment that I was not sitting in a medical school class. I would not permit myself to think: "There is nothing positive about my life right now. There is not one thing for which I am grateful." Instead, I chose even the most basic items: "I am grateful that the sun is shining. I am grateful that there are flowers on my balcony. I am grateful that I saw a hummingbird yesterday." I was already at three positive items. "I am grateful that I am alive. I am grateful that even though my legs are not working right now, at least I have legs. I am grateful for my family. I am grateful for my friends." No matter how troubling my situation seemed when

I awoke, I was always able to find some good to start my mental positive list.

My rules for the "Oh, Happy Day" game:

> *Get up everyday and start with a mental positive list of that which you are grateful. Instead of saying, "My ___ hurts" start by saying, "I am thankful that I have ____.*

The "Oh, Happy Day" game is similar to the "reframe exercise" talked about in Chapter 11 about *il malocchio*. The reframe exercise is focused more on the concept of having the ability to control your thoughts and as a result change your attitude about a particular situation. With "Oh, Happy Day" the concept is focused on starting each day by building a fortress of positive attitude so that as you move through your day all your interactions are protected from negative thoughts—how you feel about yourself, how you treat others, how others perceive you, how you perceive your relationship to the universe.

After playing the "Oh, Happy Day" game each morning picture yourself surrounded by an old stone fortress. Above one of the grey brick turrets flies a yellow flag with the black smiley face symbol. Hung above the drawbridge is a banner hung with the phrase, "Oh, Happy Day!" No one can penetrate your positive attitude fortress with negative, not even your own thoughts.

I want to explain the phrase: "How you perceive your relationship to the universe." How do you view your current situation? Do you view it as hostile or bad in some way? Is it someone else's fault you are in the situation? Do you view yourself as having any ability to change the situation?

In my observations as a person with chronic illnesses and as one who has listened to many people with disabilities, I believe two of the greatest but avoidable obstacles to healing exist when you blame your health situation on someone else and/or you see yourself as a victim.

How do you know if you are predisposed to these detrimental obstacles? Take the opportunity to listen to what comes out of your mouth. Are your utterances similar to any of these?

> "My husband's stubbornness and ill-temper all these years caused my heart attack."
>
> "I had to deal with my daughter's oppositional defiance the whole time she was growing up. Alcohol is the only way to deal with that kind of daily stress. That it why I started to drink so heavily."
>
> "My wife was too lazy to cook good meals. She always brought junk food into the house so that is why I weigh this much. It is her fault I have diabetes and osteoarthritis."

Blame your current addiction or health situation on someone else and you have shucked any personal responsibility for it. You have also relinquished all responsibility for improving your health situation. How does it serve you to blame your addiction or ill health on someone else? As discussed in Chapter 11, YOU are the person with control over making choices and acting on improvements in your life. Gather the courage to take responsibility for your health and act on that responsibility instead of blaming your ill health on someone or something else.

I realize that an event may have occurred that caused you to be blind, paralyzed or debilitated by scarring. But the event is over now. Your situation is present. The time to move from blame into self-help is now! Being stuck in blame blinds you from seeing your options for healing and acting on those opportunities. As stated earlier, there is always an aspect of your health situation over which YOU can take charge.

If you believe you are a victim, you believe yourself helpless. Believing yourself helpless extinguishes hope. Hope is the life-ring tossed out to you to grasp and pull yourself to safety from raging waters. The victim role is lethal. Stay in the victim role and you will drown. Ask yourself what is it about the victim role that serves you? Is it so that others will feel sorry for you or so that you can feel sorry for yourself? *"Fo getta bout it!" Coraggio!*

I was fortunate because Nonna, with her *testadura* stubbornness, always chose the role of fighter rather than victim. I can picture her, when faced with a daunting situation, her face motionless, her deep set eyes darkened as if in a trance. I knew she was pleading with *Dio* (God) and imploring intercession from the Madonna and her favored saints for them to give her the courage to face the situation and to show her the way. It was with that same trance-like stance that Nonna would whisper to me, *"Coraggio, Leeza. Coraggio."*

Embedded in those words were the life lessons Nonna taught me. I think back on the fact that the doctor had told a young, twenty year old, full of life, vigor and determination to conquer the world of medicine: "You will not fulfill your dream of becoming a doctor."

Thank God I had Nonna's encouragement. Thank God I still had some adolescent rebellion to prove the doctor wrong. And thank God for witnessing Nonna's choice time and again to be a *testadura* (stubborn) fighter instead of a victim. Had I to be a victim I would have accepted the role of cripple that the doctor had chosen for me and been in the institution he had prognosticated.

NEVER let another person tell you that you cannot do something or achieve something you desire. Never let someone tell you how sick you are going to be with a serious and chronic disease without telling you all the options for how healthy you can be.

Emily Dickinson got it when she wrote these eloquently encouraging words:

I dwell in possibilities
A fairer house than prose
More numerous of windows
Superior for doors

With courage you can:

- Start each day with a positive attitude.
- Dwell in the possibilities surrounding you.
- Build an impenetrable fortress of self-love.

CHAPTER 33

The Importance of Cleaning Out Emotional Baggage to Clear the Path to Loving Yourself

CAN AN ESSAY A DAY KEEP ASTHMA OR ARTHRITIS AT BAY? ETERNALLY interested in the mind-body connection, the *New York Times* title caught my attention. The story told of a study from the *Journal of the American Medical Association,* in April 1999, that followed 70 patients who were instructed to write about "the most stressful event they had ever undergone." For at least 20 minutes, on three consecutive days, the patients had to describe their "deepest thoughts and feelings" related to the traumatic experience. A control group was instructed to write about a more emotionally benign subject—their plans for that day. The doctors for all the patients were prevented from knowing whether their patients were in the trauma journaling or the control groups.

After four months, of the patients who journaled about their most stressful event, 47 percent showed improvement in their condition, 49 percent showed no change, and 4.3 demonstrated worsening of their condition. Among the patients who wrote out their plans for the day, only 24 percent showed improvement, 54 percent showed no change and 22 percent exhibited worsening of symptoms. The researchers noted that patients who went through a process of writing about a stressful event were more likely to improve or show no deterioration of their condition when worsening could have been expected. They concluded that the mind and body are interconnected and that writing about traumatic events improved the symptoms of chronic asthma and rheumatoid arthritis patients.

Dr. David Speigel, Professor and Associate Chairman of Psychiatry and Behavioral Sciences at Stanford University, commented on the findings in an editorial appearing along with the study wherein he pointed out that modern medicine treats physical conditions with disassociation from any connection to the mind.

The journaling article mirrored my experience with the effect of emotional status on my autoimmune inflammatory status. I tried my own experiment. Sitting with my eyes closed in a quiet place, I gave myself permission to spend as much time as needed and journeyed back through my memories to traumatic emotional episodes. As I relived a particular memory, a physical feeling of tightening started to constrict my chest.

It is okay now. That event in your life has passed and finished. Everything is in order now. Let go of the emotional tension you attached to it and buried within.

I visualized myself washing away the trauma with a warm cleanse of self-love and self-care. I visualized my chest freely expanding and felt the loosening from bonds of ancient injury. It was astonishing that after completing the arduous task of processing and tossing a deeply scarring memory, a path was cleared for another memory that needed healing to burst into my awareness. A calcified, decrepit scar unwelcomingly occupied precious space in my mind and perhaps in the memory of my body's cells. The festering wound's recalcitrant vagrancy pushed away room for the inner peace and cleanliness I needed to love myself and to unconditionally love others.

When the expanse of my mind is filled with equanimity, there is no room for hurt. *When I exist with a mind free of hurt I experience a body free of hurt.*

The *Essay a Day* study also supports my philosophy of having at least one confidante with whom I am able to confide and from whom I receive a supportive boost. A positive release in a safe environment is one way I maintain an emotionally clean space.

Nonna became my confidante when later in life her health problems became more significant. She held a similar philosophy as mine: Do not dwell on your health issues via spewing them onto whomever might listen. "Why should everybody have to listen to my complaints?" she would say. "Everyone has their own problems; they do not want to hear mine. I don't want to bother everyone."

For Nonna and me there was safety in knowing that we both had pain, frustration with health care, and struggles of living alone with limitations due to disability. We held a secret pact and we could confess our hardships to each other. It was understood that the expressions of pain or frustration were not complaining, rather an ability to get them off our chests. Our pact also served to boost each other's morale instead of leading each other down a pitying plunge.

Nonna and I talked nearly everyday. Upon greeting one another the first thing we would ask was, *"Come stai"* (How are you?). The answer was usually *"Bene!"* (Good!). *"Cosi, cosi"* (so, so) was code for "not so well; let's talk about it if that's okay with you." When in the presence of others, *"Cosi, cosi"* stood for "Let's talk about it later when we are alone."

Through Nonna's example, I learned how to use courage to strengthen myself emotionally so I did not waste precious energy spilling my illness woes on every ear in audio range and to know when I should share a concern so it would not fester within.

With courage you can:

- Process and purge stored resentment, anger and other emotional baggage.
- Recognize and resolve conflict instead of accumulating resentment, anger and assorted emotional baggage.

CHAPTER 34

Importance of Reducing Fear to Increase Love

I WAS IN MY TWENTIES WHEN I FIRST READ *LOVE IS LETTING GO OF FEAR* by Gerald G. Jampolsky. At that time I didn't know what the title meant. Nonetheless, Jampolsky's proposition made a lot of sense: We carry fears and resentments that can hold us back from living full and happy lives.

The book's message prompted me to take a long, close look within to uncover fears and resentments, and work at releasing those fears and practicing forgiveness, the goal being to lead a happier and healthier life. The book was a tremendous positive influence on the formation of my young conscience and I distributed many copies to family and friends. I still have my original 1981 copy to this day, so significant is the sentiment held within its yellowed musty pages.

Practicing forgiveness was the most difficult for me. I was of the same genetic stock as the Calabrese *testadura* and the same familial influence of Nonna Testadura Gigliotti. Forgiveness comes hard for the hard-headed.

As I read the book, I was saddened by regret that I had not focused on the forgiveness aspect of self-love before my mother's accidental death. Even though my mother and I had openly discussed my cache of resentment toward her and I had finally admitted its existence, I had not provided an ounce of forgiveness to her even when she openly begged forgiveness of me. That realization was not a proud moment in my life. In fact, if I allowed myself to think about it, negative thoughts about my actions would be intense enough to compel instant lament born of disdain for my foolishness, stubbornness, the pain I inflicted, and the missed opportunity to heal a paramount relationship.

Why did I have to learn the forgiveness lesson in such a devastating and permanent way?

The reality was that my mother may have taken into eternity hurt I inflicted and I loathed myself for my part in that probability. But self-loathing worked against the concept of reversing my body's attack against itself. Thus, after my mother's death I vowed to stray from the path of stockpiling unforgiveness.

As I shoveled off layers of unforgiveness muck, I began to feel lighter and happier inside. Some of the encrusted unforgivens seemed insignificant once I reached them and I took a fresh look.

Why had I held onto them for so long? How much emotional energy had I wasted confining the hoard?

I was careful not to build a new pile of resentment. It became freeing to work through conflicts so there was a resolution rather than resentment. It certainly seemed a lot less stressful to employ passive-aggressiveness and hoist the resulting resentment onto a heap in my psyche. But that meant I had to carry it around, which required a lot more energy than to deal with the conflict when it occurred, so as not to reach the resentment stage. Sometimes this meant that I set boundaries. I would not be taken advantage of or allow myself to be treated abusively. I had too much love and respect for myself to allow that. If an offender's apology was contrite and intended no future offense, forgiveness was mine to give.

The more I let go of past resentments, the more room I had inside to feel joy. I liked the new lighter, happier me. I had a lot more love and joy to give others without the big pile of unhappiness weighing down my emotional energy.

Jampolsky's issue of releasing fear was easier. To me, there were different "fear thresholds." It appeared that some people had a lower fear threshold; being afraid of the dark meant they did not go into their basement at night to do laundry; being afraid of bugs meant they did not explore the outdoors.

I had stood up against the fear of my own mortality when I was twenty. At first I was weak-kneed, but after realizing the chink in armor was self-pity, I squared off against fear, hands on hips, nose to nose, unblinking, and I won. I am not exactly sure how you measure victory against fear but I know that I did not allow it to hold me back from at least pushing headstrong toward my aspirations.

I also believed in a distinction between rational fear and irrational fear, although I was never sure who was supposed to be the line judge for deciding when fear crossed the line from rational to irrational. I believed fear was rational if it was based on fact or sound reason and prevented harm. An example was my Hungarian Grandfather Nagypapa's decision to leave his Onga, Hungary estate in 1945. In the days before his departure, the invading Nazi's were advancing toward his home from the East and the liberator Russians were advancing from the West. In his memoir Nagypapa wrote of the dreary fateful morning he and his stable hand, Joska, prepared the *szeker* (horse-drawn wood cart) for departure.

> *Joska came at dawn and woke me. We hitched the horses. It was one of those cold and damp October mornings when the air is saturated with humidity to the point that the rain begins to form right around you. The makeshift canvas canopy over the szeker was saturated stiff by the rain but watertight. I wordlessly shook hands with Joska, climbed up, and off I was. As I turned left at our gatepost, I couldn't resist the temptation Lot's wife felt a couple thousand years ago and tried to catch a last glimpse back. But the canopy prevented me of doing so, which was just as well.*

After Nagypapa reluctantly fled his beloved yet besieged motherland, there were fellow countrymen who accused him of being a coward.

From the books and articles I have read about World War I and World War II, not only could you be assured death and destruction from the invaders, but the so-called liberators often pillaged to a worse degree than the invaders.

My grandfather had lived through World War I as a preteen. Unfortunately, his young eyes and ears had witnessed obliterating destruction, unnatural death and the brutal, repeated raping of an innocent villager woman. Now as a wealthy landowner, husband and father of two young daughters, he had the responsibility to decide whether to stay or to leave his embattled homeland. Nagypapa had no idea whether they would be injured, homeless or starve to death in an attempt to flee, but he had the courage to try against what he believed would happen if he remained in Onga. I am sure that fear was embedded in viewing either scenario.

Nagypapa had his personal war experiences to enliven the fears, but he also had wisdom. He was an incredibly wise man by nature, but he kept himself informed through literature and dialogue with both colleagues of his educated class and members of the working class. I believe his decision to shield his beautiful wife and young daughters was based on wisdom and facts. I believe it was also based on rational fear. Nagypapa gathered courage, the sum of which must have been more tremendous than I can imagine, packed a horse cart and left.

The Barczay estate in Onga was confiscated and eventually destroyed; never again would a Barczay possess the estate or land. But, his "precious girls", as he referred to them, wife Annie, young Anna and sweet blonde-curled, blue-eyed Julia (my mother) never came to harm.

I try to balance the scales of fear when making important decisions. An issue which has caused great consternation when trying to sort through what might be irrational fear is my decision-making about whether to utilize new medications or medical treatments. I have heard confessions from friends of their similar struggle. Their physician suggests the use of a different medication. They read the medication package insert, research the drug on the Internet and listen to comments from others. There is the inclination to focus on and lock onto the worst side-effects listed, some as devastating as death, suicide and impotency. They lock onto "frightening facts mode", resulting in *fear*. The outweighing many ways the medication might help are disregarded or thwarted by fear. I am not being critical. When the immunosuppressive agent Methotrexate was suggested by both my neurologist and rheumatologist, I found myself in a similar rational versus irrational balancing act.

Methotrexate was reported in a lot of medical literature to be effective in treating rheumatoid arthritis. There was scarce medical literature to support the use of Methotrexate for myasthenia gravis, but enough for the Neurology Fellow and Department Chair to support its use in my case to kill two disease birds with one stone. I was given the quick doctor-office explanation of the serious side effects. Continuing in my pre-med mode, I did more in-depth study of the drug on my own. The chemical's intent once inside the body was to find and kill fast-reproducing cells and destroy without discriminating between good cells or bad cells. The drug was also used for treating cancer, but as a chemotherapy agent it was given in much greater strength than dosages for treating rheumatoid arthritis. Even so, the side effects for the lower dosage contained foreboding words like life-threatening liver damage, blood and bone marrow problems including leukemia, decreased white blood cell and platelet counts that could result in an inability to fight infection or stop bleeding, possibility of lung problems, and probability of hair loss. *Possibility of liver biopsies? Probability of hair loss? Not my thick, naturally chestnut-highlighted hair.* I already believed my gnarled hands unsightly. The last thing I wanted to do was diminish an aspect of my appearance for which I remained proud.

I filled the prescription and poured a few of its contents into the palm of my hand. The minute size of each pill was a great contrast to its tremendous potency. A tablet the size and shape of a dried orzo noodle could lead to the death and destruction of so many cells inside my body. I set the small bottle on the lace-covered top of my tall bedroom chest of drawers. I entered the room each day and looked at the bottle. *Is today the day?* Fearful thoughts flooded my pondering and overcame action.

I prolonged the advent of Methotrexate for several years. In the years between filling my first Methotrexate prescription and commencing the treatment, rheumatoid arthritis ran wild through my body, executing damage in as many joints as possible. When I finally started Methotrexate, it took the edge off the force of the arthritis army. The immobilization from fear taught me a painful lesson. Was my fear rational or irrational? Was the decision to forgo Methotrexate prudent? I am sure I could find supporters for either side.

I have not experienced any of the life-threatening side effects of Methotrexate in the twelve-plus years I have taken it. But I

suspect I could have avoided some of the irreparable joint damage the disease incurred while it was rampant, and that could
have been avoided if Methotrexate had been present to mitigate.

I do take careful consideration to avoid serious infection,
reducing my immunosuppressive agents until the infection sub-
sides. I try to be vigilant about going for blood lab checks every
six weeks; I never miss yearly mammograms and pelvic exams;
and seek other skin or tissue checks if any body occurrence
appears suspicious. I avoid infection-ridden situations and constantly sanitize my hands, but I do not let it rise to fanaticism.
I have minor hair loss and notice an increase in the brown strands
in my brush when I increase my dose of Methotrexate, but I balance any paranoia by listening to friends who have had similar
experiences while pregnant or entering menopause.

I am informed of the risks associated with taking medications, but I use that information to be vigilant, not to dwell on the
negative. It is very easy to read nausea and headache as a listed
side effect and imagine that my stomach hurts or my skull feels
pressure. I refuse that line of thinking now. My focus now is not
on fear from the harm the medication may cause. The research
is important so that I know for what to pay attention. Instead of
fear I take a big gulp of courage, swallow or inject the drug and
say a prayer that it does the maximum good I need it to while
being protected from the dangers.

The same philosophy for making medical treatment decisions can be extrapolated to other important life decisions. Take
a gulp of courage and you may find the fear dispensed after you
step forward.

But what if you are truly afraid?

I visit my sister Laura and her family often, despite the fact
that there is a 90-minute commute between our homes. One of
the long-drive consolations is that my sister packs me a parting
gift of sentimental precious Italian or Hungarian food treats to
nibble during the trip back home. If you are Italian you understand

the parting food package, just in that off-chance that I get stranded in the metropolis of Detroit or the farmlands encompassing Lansing and would need food to survive. On one of my recent trips home, my sister placed the food bag handle around my wrist and pressed a Joyce Meyer lecture on cassette into my palm. She encouraged me to listen to Joyce Meyer to pass the drive time from her home to mine. The lecture was titled *Free Indeed* and it was about freedom from fear and dread. I popped in the tape as soon as I reached the corner of her street. I was immediately engaged in Joyce's comments about how fear can keep us from doing what we are called to do in our days, and even bigger, in our life.

My thoughts drifted from Joyce's message to a recent conversation I had with my cousin Stephen about fear. We had commented about how we may have a deeply seated fear that is not recognizable even to our reflective and honest selves. Our conversation had turned to how the unrecognized fears had influenced inaction in our lives, despite both of being self-motivated, ambitious people. My brain segued into a discussion my brother Paul and I had regarding fear of success issues. I was jolted back to Joyce's commanding voice as part of my brain picked up her telling a story about a woman who was afraid to drive a car on the freeway.

Joyce, in typical fiery manner shouted, "Do it afraid!"

I leaned closer to the speakers in the dashboard to make sure I had heard correctly. "Do it afraid!"

At first her comment struck me as being harsh. Then I thought about the point Joyce was making about fear and dread: we need to be free of fear and dread in order to move forward in life and do what it is we need to do. I believe that what we need to do may not be as extravagant as moving to a third-world country and saving sick babies. But we may need to free ourselves so that we can heal. Whether that healing is physical, emotional, spiritual, if we hold ourselves back out of fear, the healing may be blocked. Joyce's suggestion to "Do it afraid!" made a lot of sense.

You may be afraid; you may not be able to resolve the fear or dread, so you might as well do it afraid. The alternative is to not do it at all. But in your inaction, you are not moving forward and you continue to be stuck in fear and dread mode.

What about those who are "afraid" to let others know they are afraid? Joyce Meyer went on to say that some people carry around fear in a "hidden bag" so that others do not see it. They may go on with the strong, macho-guy face, but it takes a lot of energy to hide fear and it sometimes leaks out in unpleasant behaviors, such as control and manipulation. Joyce alerted me of the need to be free of the fear and dread of those who manipulate us. The irony, she points out, is that those who manipulate or oppress us are often acting out of their own fears.

I think about Stephen, Paul, and me and our suppressed or otherwise unrecognized fears and how difficult it is to discover those fears, the courage it takes to admit those fears to others, and the courage it takes to act to overcome those fears.

Have the courage to move forward in a way that can influence a better outcome for you and your life than if you had not moved forward at all. It may be difficult to move forward but self-respect will be garnered in that movement. Not only will you be doing what it is you need to do with your life, but you will also grow in love for who you are and how you live your life.

With *courage* you can:
- Distinguish between rational and irrational fear
- Discover the fear that blocks you from receiving and giving love.
- "Do it afraid" or face and blast through the fear that blocks you from receiving and giving love.

CHAPTER 35

The Importance of Humor in Loving Yourself

In 1964, NORMAN COUSINS WAS THE EDITOR OF SATURDAY REVIEW. RETURNING home from an overseas trip he felt the flu-like symptoms of fever and aches. Within a week the symptoms had progressed and he could barely move his neck, arms, hands, fingers and legs. He was hospitalized and diagnosed as having ankylosing spondylitis, a type of arthritis where the joints of the spine (the vertebrae) become inflamed. It has a reputation of becoming a chronic and debilitating disease.

One way to measure inflammation is by using a blood test that calculates the sedimentation rate of blood cells in a test tube. A high sedimentation rate indicates a level of inflammation somewhere in the body. The normal sedimentation rate for men is 0–15 millimeters per hour. At hospitalization, Norman Cousins' sedimentation rate was over 80 millimeters per hour. His pain was severe. But he was determined to not allow the disease to progress and to not accept the disease as chronic.

Mr. Cousins said he could deal with the pain as long as he knew he was working to help his body recover. He let the doctors run their course of medical treatment in the hospital and decided to run his own attack on the disease, what he called "the full exercise of the affirmative emotions as a factor in enhancing body chemistry." In other words, he would use laughter as his medical treatment regimen.

Alan Funt, the producer of the television show *Candid Camera*, sent to Cousins' hospital room clips from his funniest shows and a projector to view the program. Marx Brothers films were also added to Cousins' show time. "I made the joyous discovery that ten minutes of genuine belly laughter had an anesthetic effect and would give me at least two hours of pain-free sleep," said Cousins. "When the pain-killing effect of the laughter wore off, we would switch on the motion-picture projector again, and not infrequently, it would lead to another pain-free sleep interval."

Cousins found the positive effect of laughter on his feelings of wellbeing so interesting he had blood tests performed to determine whether there were actual corresponding physiological changes. He had his blood work checked directly before a laughter episode and then four hours after. What was revealed was astounding! There was a drop in the sedimentation rate of at least five points after each laughing session "I was greatly elated by the discovery that there is a physiological basis for the ancient theory that laughter is good medicine," he said.

Each day, Cousins slowly recovered and when he returned to work at the *Saturday Review* he was free of the potential chronic illness.

My mother discovered Norman Cousins' proclamation of laughter as good medicine and excitedly provided me a copy of his book. Always the scientist, I was fascinated by such a blatant example of the mind-body connection. My mother decided to utilize it with her own twist. We were both lovers of music, dance, and beauty. She rented or borrowed videotapes of every known musical motion-picture. She helped me into my wheelchair, wheeled me into the living room, and there in front of our old 19-inch color television set we would become caught up in the transforming world of song, dance and the inevitable happy ending where love prevailed Both of us vocalists, singing aloud during the movies was permitted and often performed over the volume of the television set. We laughed until we cried. Sometimes the laughter was a result of a comedic script, other times from the sheer corniness of the decades-old film. I was not only lightening my spirit with laughter, I was flooding my senses with that which brought me joy: music, dance and laughter.

Humor can sometimes be the only effective method of breaking the tension in unbearably humiliating medical situations. I could make myself miserable with mortification or I could laugh at the uncomfortable circumstances. That meant laughing at *myself,* which made it easier on me and for everyone who had to provide care for me in the embarrassing situation. It was humor that made an awful circumstance an entertaining and thus bearable occasion.

I am grateful to have experienced the healing power of humor in many contexts. As unlikely as it may appear, I try to find the courage to use humor to help me through a difficult situation. But if I am in a prolonged period of acute pain and feeling emotionally worn and tired from the inability to get uninterrupted sleep, it is difficult to feel humor or utter a chuckle.

In India, Dr. Madan Kataria started what he termed "Laughter Yoga: A Global Movement for Health, Joy and World Peace." Laughter yoga combines laughter with yogic breathing practices.

Dr. Kataria believes that 15 to 30 minutes of laughter a day enhances the circulation of oxygen in the body, facilitates movement of organs and releases pent-up stress. He commends the results of deep laughter for increasing immune health. You can check it out on his website at www.laughteryoga.org. You can also catch laughter yoga clips on youtube.com.

It takes courage to laugh when the pain in your body is flamed by tongues of fire you know come straight from hell.

Dr. Kataria says he encourages those who do not feel as if they can laugh, to "fake it until you make it". Stand in front of the mirror. Make a wrinkled, grumpy face and laugh at how ridiculous your face looks or how ridiculous you believe you are standing there trying to make yourself laugh. And then laugh. Fake it; force it. Try the soundless belly laugh. Try the high-pitched, shrilly Wicked Witch of the West laugh. If you have the courage to at least try to laugh before you know it, you may end up with a chuckle and experience the laughter benefits.

With courage you can:

- Find humor in every challenging situation.
- Use humor to heal.
- Use humor to get through an intense pain episode.
- Perfect the ability to laugh at yourself.

CHAPTER 36

The Importance of Life Purpose as a Key Component of Self-Love

From as far back as I can recall it gave my life purpose to help others. I was the consummate Girl Scout, serving through my young years from Brownie to Senior Scout. The drive to help others as a doctor had provided the fortitude to finish pre-med studies despite tremendous health obstacles.

But after I graduated and was applying to medical schools, rheumatoid arthritis continued raging its vicious war against my body. I now needed the full-time use of a wheelchair and was little more than confined to bed. The medical school application required a written recommendation from my academic major's department head. I called the chairwoman of the Biology Department, and respecting her distinguished position and valuable time, got straight to my request for a medical school recommendation.

After a long, weighty silence, she took a serious and uncomfortable-sounding breath. "How is your health? I heard you are having a difficult time, now having to use a wheelchair. Is that true?"

"Yes," was my short response followed by another long silence.

I heard her take another deep breath, this one sounding more deliberate. She said she was reluctant to forward her recommendations because she believed the rigors of medical school would be too demanding for my physical condition.

I tried to grasp the reality of her words. *I can't believe she is reluctant to write my recommendations.* She was a mentor. I had always admired the dignified and professional manner in which she sought to impart science education, to conduct her own research and pound the door of the National Institutes of Health for grants to improve the college's science program. She had been the faculty member responsible for my selection as the Mount St. Mary's College Excellence in Biological Sciences Award recipient, less than one year prior. I was stunned.

I argued that I was determined and I believed I could finish medical school. *She knows you are determined. She watched you limp and drag your pain-stricken body through the last year of undergrad.* But maybe that was it. She had watched me limp and drag myself to the graduation finish line. I tried to focus on her viewpoint instead of falling into resentment. *She believes she is acting in your best interest.* But my lifelong dream was to go to medical school and this single act of withholding a recommendation could block the way to my goal.

Okay God. You know my motivation to become a doctor is so I can help others through the medical arts. I ferociously battled through significant health challenges to finish pre-med schooling. Now why the med school application barrier? Why did you give me the drive, intellect and compassion to be a healer, yet there are all these physical and procedural roadblocks? What do you want me to do now?

Realistically, what could I do? You could say I was one of those people who actually felt her calling deep in her core. I had always felt fortunate that I had such clarity of purpose. *But what now?*

I spent some of the fragile, stiff and pain-forced bed hours reading about medical missionaries, stoking the blazing fire of passion within me to become a doctor. I knew myself well enough to realize that I felt my best when I was helping or bringing serenity and happiness to others. Living my life with purpose was key to self-love.

But what about the roadblocks to living my life with purpose? The answer was simply a matter of figuring out how to overcome or sidestep the roadblocks. I refused to turn back or plop myself on the ground in defeat. As various roadblocks appeared in my path, I followed an analytical approach to overcome them. Do I hurdle or sidestep? What technique should I use? What do I need to succeed? What do I already possess to help me succeed?

To discover the solution for the medical school roadblock I took stock of what I possessed. I had intellect and motivation. I recognized that empathy was an element of the passion I had for doctoring. I was an empathetic listener, having some training as a peer counselor in high school and undergrad, having received affirming feedback from numerous hours of listening.

And then I came up with a solution. I could attend Master's Degree classes in Marriage, and Family Therapy even from my wheelchair. I could conduct a therapy practice from a wheelchair if necessary while regaining my strength and fortitude to attend medical school. With my good grades and undergrad science and psychology emphasis I would have no problem getting accepted into a Master's Degree program.

I registered for Marriage and Family Therapy program classes at California State University at Northridge (CSUN) and moved into an apartment close enough to campus for the wheelchair accessible van to transport me in my wheelchair to classes.

I enjoyed one psychology professor in particular, Dr. C. He was to me the classic professor/therapist—grey hair, balding at the top but long enough on the sides and back to display waves of liberalism, compassionately soft spoken and funny. His therapy focus was on relationship issues, an area for which I, too, had enthusiasm. But as we got into practicum, I found it difficult to listen to a person who was struggling emotionally because she found her life was monotonous. This was a person with a loyal husband, healthy children and home in beautiful San Fernando Valley, California. I, on the other hand, had my entire family unit killed in a car accident the year before, was unmarried with no children, had legs that did not work and was not in medical school. I struggled to develop more compassion for people who I believed should be happy and grateful because they appeared to have everything, and I chastised myself for my lack of empathy.

I did, however, love interacting with people struggling with health, terminal illness and grieving issues. I transferred to the hospital chaplain program at the University of Michigan Mott Children's Hospital. *What intensity!* Pain and death at the door-step of children, their parents and their families. I felt the importance of my work every moment within the hospital. And I was thrilled to be functioning within a hospital, emboldening my desire to get to medical school. The hospital chaplain experiences would help me in my interaction with patients when I became a doctor.

But soon however, I found myself besieged with feelings of inadequacy. Angry parents demanded to know why God was causing their child to suffer. The frightened look in the large, dark eyes of children, against their emaciated, blanched faces, pierced through me seeking reassurance. But I failed to adequately respond. I did not have the answers to why children suffer; to why innocent infants die. *God, please give me some direction as to what you want me to do with this life you've given me.*

At the same time, my brother Paul was in his first year of law school and he repeatedly urged me to join him.

"A lawyer? I don't want to be *lawyer!*" I spoke with disdain as if lawyers were despicable creatures.

Paul, born with a true lawyer's wit and tongue, argued that a law degree could open a world of opportunity to help people receive good health care and to influence the health care field.

Money was not a motivator. The first job I accepted after law school was for $27,000 per year. The entire year's salary was less than the total of my law school loans. My law school friend Donna emphatically urged me to reject the offer. She reasoned that I could not live off the poverty-level salary, especially with the hefty monthly law school loans obligation.

But for me, it was always about believing I was fulfilling a life purpose. I was a kid who knew to the core of my bones that I would become a doctor. When serious physical roadblocks prevented medical school entry it was complicated to sort and decipher what my life purpose was. In order to see clearly, I had to tease away my strong emotional attachment to being a doctor. I told myself not to abandon the doctor dream, but rather to set it aside for the time being.

I took inventory of my education, skills and talents. But there was still something missing. *What is it that makes a job a vocation? What gives the spark to life purpose?*

I sat without distraction, eyes closed. *Recall a time you felt excited inside. What was the event that brought you excitement?* I lingered in the memory until all of the internal and external elements of that moment in time came back to life. I saw what I had been wearing. I sensed the heat generated from my adrenalin-enhanced exuberance. I felt the tightness of the corners of my mouth as I smiled in fulfillment. I envisioned the light that emitted from my eyes, sprung forth from a soul heartened by knowing it had helped a fellow human being. *What was it about the interaction that provoked the feeling of excitement? What aspects of the experience harvested fulfillment? What actions are meaningful and bring a sense of helping others?*

I used the deeper reflection application of senses exercise to recall other times in my life of distinct happiness. I went back again in my mind to taste, smell, hear and feel experiences of fulfillment and joy-giving. The more deeply and honestly I reflected on life experiences and attached feelings, the clearer the picture became of where to head with my life's purpose.

I realized that there were core principles to what I believed were my life purpose. Astoundingly, these core principles were not solely applicable to doctoring. Hands-on helping vulnerable people, serving with joy, kindness, compassion and love could fit into many careers. It seems so obvious and simple to me now, but I was so entrenched in my own idea of what my life purpose should be I could not see it then.

Whether I am speaking to a high school career day class, first-year law students or anyone else who might be struggling with the fundamental question, "What is my purpose on earth?" my message is it is yours to discover. Take inventory of your strengths or ask for feedback on what others believe are your strengths. Quiet your mind and reflect on occasions that fostered feelings of fulfillment or a sense of accomplishing good. Combine your strengths and what you know brings you fulfillment into core principles to form your life purpose. You will find that you can perform your everyday job and your family obligations as a vocation no matter how insignificant or monotonous they may seem. And as you live each day honoring your life purpose, self-love and self-respect flourish.

I had no idea there were legal careers devoted to advocating for people with disabilities. But my life purpose core principles were a perfect match. I could pour forth my wealth of compassion with hands-on application and at the same time use my medical training and law school education.

Surging feelings of purpose and fulfillment took me by surprise as I performed a job for which I was paid! I was helping vulnerable people, assisting them to advocate for what they needed to be independent and hence feel the fulfillment of living their own life purpose. I was helping parents of severely disabled kids obtain medically necessary treatment or life-sustaining treatment in the home instead of in a hospital or institutional setting.

To the reality that rheumatoid arthritis sucked stamina and oppressed body movement, to the fact that I was a legal novice elbowing my way into federal courtrooms and corporate lawyers' offices, I could only cry, *Coraggio! You want to help people ... here you are. Now get moving.*

Friends and family remarked that not even perfectly healthy people could have kept the physical and emotional pace I had for the work I loved so much. But that was the lesson. The more fulfilling the task, the more on point with my life purpose, the more energy I had. Sure I had a lot of physical limitations that limited me in other ways, but my physical and emotional stamina was at peak when I believed and felt I was fulfilling my life purpose.

I had a similar life purpose experience a few years later when I accepted the position of Michigan Senate Policy Advisor for children, family and health issues. In quiet reflection, I applied my life purpose core principle to what I knew of the policy advisor position. *God, help me know this is the right direction and grant me courage.* It felt like a perfect fit. I was advocating a position to help vulnerable people even though my job tasks were dissimilar to my staff attorney position. I could not have imagined that identifying and applying my life purpose core principles could work for such diverse job titles. Yet there I was, in the middle of state senators as they went about drafting proposed legislation to help children, families and medically fragile people in Michigan.

During my senate policy advisor stint some of the most controversial issues to hit the Michigan Legislature erupted. I was assigned to the legislative maneuverings surrounding the hot button cloning, assisted suicide, partial-birth abortion, foster care program revamp, shift to managed care for Medicaid recipients, and welfare reform. All my life experience from Girl Scouts, pre-med, pediatric hospital chaplain, Marriage and Family Therapy graduate classes, law school and disability rights attorney was used at some point. And even though I was physically and emotionally exhausted, my soul rejoiced as only a soul can when it is synced with its life purpose. *Could there ever be a more perfect match of my life experiences with my life purpose?* I should know better than to tempt fate with such a question.

The answer came amidst a gruesome perverted set of circumstances. As a policy advisor with a Juris Doctorate degree, I had been assigned as Committee Counsel to the Michigan Senate Judiciary Committee. Jack Kevorkian was on trial for having assisted to death his 30th patient. Legislation to <u>ban</u> assisted suicide had just been introduced, as was legislation that would <u>legalize</u> assisted suicide. Both bills were assigned to the Judiciary Committee. I read through hundreds of pages of draft legislation, policy arguments, and listened to proponents from each side.

When I thought about the criteria Jack Kevorkian was openly proposing for accessing assisted suicide, I realized I was a candidate for assisted suicide at that very moment and in my current situation. Disregard the fact I did not have a terminal illness, was highly educated and alert, and was employed full-time as an attorney-policy advisor for Michigan Senate. If I wanted to, under Jack Kevorkian's criteria I could get in line and have him take my life. There was something horribly wrong with that reality. What if I was not fortunate enough to have the tremendous love and support of family and friends? What if I did not have good health care? I am an overly guilt-ridden, Italian Roman-Catholic. Would I have felt guilty enough to get in the death line solely because I did not want to burden my family and friends? If I had no health care would it have been easier for me to get in the death line?

A proposal to legalize assisted suicide made its way onto the Michigan November 1998 election ballot. I wrote a monograph about my observations and experiences as a person with a disability living in an era of health care rationing, limited societal supports and negative societal biases against people with disabilities and people at the end of life. I gave sections of the monograph to anyone who wanted to use it. I began giving small group presentations about my observations and experiences. The fact that I was an attorney appeared to lend more credibility to my opinion. The word spread and I was asked to speak more frequently to larger groups. At one point I was speaking once or twice a day in different regions of Michigan or in surrounding states.

Then it hit me. Life purpose. I get it. Perhaps this is why I had to endure two chronic disabilities. I had authentic experiences regarding bias and prejudice against people with disabilities. Perhaps this is why I am a lawyer. I have a doctorate level understanding of constitutional parameters and the development and enforcement of state and federal law. Everything clicked into place for me. By having the courage to follow my heart, to undergo honest self-reflection and to heed intuition, I had converged upon life purpose. By using courage to go after the whisperings of my heart, with my life purpose core principles, I had found the joy and hope that garnered the physical stamina to make it happen. Other fruits found in the courage cornucopia manifested joy, hope, strength, fulfillment, self-esteem, self-worth and self-love.

Several months after the 1998 election, I found myself once more applying the life-purpose core principles. I contemplated leaving the Senate Policy Advisor position for an opportunity to work as staff to Governor John Engler. *It feels like a perfect match of my life-purpose core principles to job tasks. God, help me know this is the right direction and grant me courage.* I admired Governor Engler's strong stance on social issues and felt fortunate to work on those critical issues as Health and Human Services Policy Coordinator. Again, to my amazement, it was a beautiful, flourishing match. Not only was I in a position to work on policies to help families and children, and to help expand access to quality health care in the state of Michigan, collaboration with the National Governors Association meant an opportunity to work on national policy as well. Again I asked, *Could there be a more perfect match of my life experiences with my life purpose? Coraggio!*

I am grateful for the lesson of acting on what I believe is important. My soul rejoices in living out its imprinted purpose. I could never have imagined that a person like me, with limiting disabilities, could have lived so much of my life in fulfilling service. I feel fortunate for the opportunities that await me as I step out in courage. I feel appreciation for the gifts of self-worth and self-love that appear with knowing I lived a day as a good person and fulfilling the purpose of that day. I feel blessed for the inexplicable miracle of physical stamina that increases and physical pain that lessens as self-love and personal fulfillment permeate my being.

One year prior to the telephone call in which my request for a medical school recommendation was denied and I thought the denial a roadblock to my life purpose, I had had an opportunity to give advice on experiencing the joy, fulfillment and self-worth of living a life of purpose. I had stood and walked to the podium to deliver the Mount Saint Mary's College 1984 Commencement address. The podium was situated on top of the hill on which the white stucco St. Mary's Chapel stands guardian over the campus. Two flights of stone steps led below to where my fellow classmates and loved ones were seated. From where I stood high above Santa Monica I could see cloudless, bright blue sky folding into the deeper blue of the Pacific Ocean. The Southern California sun was merciless even in May, bearing down on the graduates and creating steam-baths of the long black graduation robes. Many loved ones, dressed in shirts, ties and other finery used a graduation ceremony program to stir face-cooling breezes.

"My *dear* friends," I started. I heard my amplified voice echo as it bounced through the open expanse. "If there is one gift I can leave you with this day, it is to see yourself truly as the special person you are."

The commencement message centered on using the occasion of graduation to recognize what unique qualities and talents you possess in order to carry them forth and apply them in the next endeavor.

As I think back on the commencement message, I discover the irony of how I needed to use my own commencement advice one year later to work around a life roadblock. I also realize that it was the process of recognizing what was special about me that led me to finding purpose and fulfillment. So now, more than twenty-five years later I shout again from the hilltop: Take the time and honesty to recognize what makes you special. Close your eyes and discover what excites you. What brings warmth to your soul? What makes you smile? Do not be limited to believing that you can only accomplish your life purpose through a career. One of this world's paramount life purposes is to raise a family. Life purpose can be getting up each day with resolve to be happy throughout the day and appreciating each moment of the day. Imagine how much joy you would spread to the world if your singular life purpose was to make one person smile each day.

Coraggio. Courage to see yourself truly as the special person you are. Courage to love yourself for the special person you are. Courage to act on your unique qualities and what brings you joy and fulfillment.

With courage you can:

- Sit quietly and discover the stirrings of your heart.

- Recognize and love the special person you are.

- Live the life you have been given.

- Act on your unique qualities and that which brings you joy and fulfillment.

- Meditate by lingering in memories and think about each sense as you linger in the memory. What do you recall of the sounds, tastes, smells, looks, physical sensations? What feelings were associated with the memory? Use this all-sensory recollection to help discern what actions bring you joy, fulfillment, and a sense of self-worth.

- Identify your life-purpose core principles.

- Apply your life-purpose core principles to your daily routine or new opportunity.

- Find your life purpose and *andiamo!* (go for it)

CHAPTER 37

Understanding Processed Food Cravings to Achieve Self-Loving Food Choices

I AM NOT PERFECT. I AM GRATEFUL FOR NONNA'S EXAMPLE OF COURAGE AND determination to make a life-saving dietary change, especially when I feel as if falling off the healthy diet wagon. After two decades of following a low-fat, high vegetable and fruit diet I found out I had a basal cell carcinoma on my forehead. A nickel-sized hole would have to be carved out of my skull in a location which would be noticeable. *Why another challenge to my vanity? Was not*

the surgical scars on my chest and knees enough? Were all those years of eating tofu and bean sprouts touted for reducing the likelihood of cancer for naught? I am going home to eat a whole bag of chips and to wash them down with artificially sweetened, flavored and colored lemonade! I felt discouraged!

By the time I got home I had talked myself out of the binge because I knew the physiological joint swelling and pain I would endure after ingesting salty, greasy cuisine would not be worth the moments of self-indulgent pleasure.

Temptation more often appeared when I did not feel well and processed, tasty foodstuffs seemed easy or soothing. The conundrum was that the most important time to follow a health-supporting diet was when I was not feeling well. A new acquaintance helped me understand that some of the cravings stemmed from primitive instinct and physiological reactions.

Dr. Douglas Lisle, Ph.D., explained that our DNA may continue to be coded with the food-gathering survival genes of our caveman ancestors and that calorie-dense food was preferred because food was difficult to come by in ancient times. In his book, *The Pleasure Trap*, Dr. Lisle discusses how as modern civilizations began to evolve, food gathering became more efficient. Dietary excess appeared for those high enough in social class to have adequate food supplies. Certain pleasure chemicals were released in the brain as food was ingested. As the ability for dietary excess occurred, so did the diseases of dietary excess or, as he referred to it, the "Diseases of Kings."

> *With modern food production techniques, the modern diet has shifted consistently in the direction of our innate preferences toward greater and still greater caloric density. This has resulted in the consumption of more animal products and other high-fat, high-sugar processed foods. As a result, the common man and woman now suffer from the Diseases of Kings.*

Dr. Lisle points out that traditional medicine solution to high blood pressure, high cholesterol and diabetes, is the *addition* of a medication. He observes that in the alternative healing tradition, solutions to the same disease conditions involve *subtraction.*

> *The real culprits in most modern-day health problems are excesses, not deficiencies. It is the subtraction of these excesses that will solve most of the problems, not the addition of medications or supplements. Not surprisingly, the subtraction of excess is nearly always more effective at restoring health than is the addition of anything, be it dietary supplements or medications.*

Dr. Lisle's premise supports my philosophy of using courage to balance your diet with low-fat protein and fresh vegetables, all foods eaten in moderation. With courage you can view a healthy diet from a perspective that avoids constant cravings but allows for occasional splurging; sharing salt and butter laden popcorn at the movies on Saturday night will not have the same long-term negative health effects if you followed a low-fat, fresh vegetable and fruit diet the preceding week.

Use courage to:

- Resist the momentary pleasure of caloric rich foods.
- Understand what is behind your unhealthful cravings so that you can outsmart the craving.
- Have healthful options available and a strategy in place to make it easier to fortify your body with healthful foods when you are feeling low-energy.

CHAPTER 38

Family Love and Tradition to Achieve Lifestyle Balance

I DO NOT MEAN TO PORTRAY FOOD AS THE ONLY POTENTIAL BAD FACTOR in lifestyles. A lifestyle has many aspects: food, exercise, work, and relationships with family and friends. Fundamental elements of my lifestyle and the lifestyles of my family and friends is loving, supporting and staying connected with one another. Gathering with family and friends is a vital means with which to stay connected and share tradition, love, support, problems and joys. Often food is front and center to these get-togethers. The fare may be as elaborate as the Sunday family meal or as simple as cappuccino and biscotti at a mid-point meeting cafe.

My family and I foster a lifestyle that perpetuates the culture and tradition of our Italian and Hungarian ancestors. Part of our cultural exposure involves enjoying each other's company, helping and loving each other. We espouse traditional foods and food-based traditions. Christmas Eve was the paramount event of our Christmas season, carrying forward the cultural and religious traditions of our Italian ancestors from generations past.

Nonna spent an entire week preparing the seven different types of fishes present at the celebration. First she purchased the Baccala (salted and dried cod) from Giglio's Italian store. She would soak the Baccala in water, each day discarding the old water with extracted salt from the fish curing process and adding new fresh water. When the fish was desalted enough, she prepared the white flaky filets as two separate dishes, one breaded and fried, and one slow-baked in a bath of thick tomato and garlic sauce.

Next she would fill the kitchen sink with water in an attempt to thaw the ten pound block of *calamari* (squid), also purchased from Giglio's Italian store. Once thawed, each of the flaccid calamari needed to be beheaded and then stripped by hand of its guts, very carefully to avoid its purple dye from staining clothes or counters. The process took hours; hence as the oldest granddaughter I was recruited to assist. To my disgust, my hands would smell for days like rotted fish, no matter with what I scrubbed them or with what strong scented lotion I tried to disguise the stench. Care had to be taken throughout the rigorous process in order to maintain the animal's rubbery tube shape for stuffing with breadcrumbs. The stuffed calamaris were then baked. Nonna prepared a second calamari dish by cutting the tubes crosswise into thick rings that were pan fried in Italian breadcrumbs.

Pesce a la Padella (smelt) my grandfather had caught in Lake Huron during the smelt season were brought up from the downstairs deep-freezer and thawed. The fish were decapitated before lightly breaded and fried.

Pasta sarde (anchovy spaghetti) was much simpler to prepare. Cloves of fresh garlic were lightly browned in olive oil, adding a menacing dose of anchovy paste, and stirring the mixture into a thick ceramic bowl of steaming spaghetti. Spaghetti with a tomato clam sauce added up to seven fish dishes. Thanks be to God Nonna was superstitious of snakes and eels, thus we were spared having to eat the eel that our *cugini* (cousins) did on Christmas Eve.

As we gathered at the Christmas Eve table, the origins of the seven fish Southern Italian Christmas Eve meal tradition was discussed. It was the *Cena della Vigilia,* the wait for the miraculous birth of Christ in which Catholics from centuries past fasted on Christmas Eve until after receiving communion at the Vigil Mass. In more modern times it was *La Vigilia di Natale* (Christmas Eve), a Catholic holiday of abstinence from eating meat. The number seven symbolized the seven sacraments of the Catholic Church, the seven gifts of the Holy Spirit, the seven days it took Mary and Joseph to ride from Jerusalem to Bethlehem, and the number representing God. Nonna also told us the number seven meant the Biblical reference to the total number of loaves and fishes (five fish and two loaves) with which Jesus performed a miracle to feed the hundreds who gathered to hear his Sermon on the Mount.

In any event, seven fishes were seven too many for my sister and me. Each year we would attempt to be unnoticed in the lack of fishy entrees on our dinner plate, splurging later at the Italian Christmas cookie table. An entire card table was devoted to the piles of delicate flat pizzelle disks that reminded me of lace doilies, frosted "S" anise-flavored cookies, and my favorite pignolata (terdelli), small pieces of fried dough coated with thick honey that adhered small pieces of crushed cinnamon stick and finely chopped chocolate.

Our Easter dinner tradition was the Pascal lamb and *Pane di Pasqua* (Easter bread). Nonna would braid the risen anise-sweetened yeast dough into a ring shape the size of a baking sheet. Delicately woven between the bread braids was a colorful hard-boiled egg for each family member. After baking, the masterfully contoured, colorful bread was frosted with a white glaze. Year after year, this symbol continued to make our eyes light up and our hearts happy as we entered from Easter morning Mass to see it adorning the center of the Easter table.

At the multi-generational family gatherings of my childhood, we would raise a glass of Grandpa Francesco's wine and join him in offering an enthusiastic toast of *"Salute!"* (To your health). At the table with all generations present we would hear the stories of courage and tradition. We could speak our truth, and experience the love and support of family.

To Nonna's mealtime urging of *"Mangia!"* I add the phrase *"salute"* and thus combine my grandparents' favorite mealtime utterances to urge you to *"Mangia bene salute!"* (Eat well to your good health.)

Use courage to:

- Make time *a mangiare* (to eat) meals with family and friends.
- Discover ways to prepare healthy versions of traditional, sentimental, cultural, favorite foods.
- Find a way to introduce healthy versions of sentimental family foods in traditional family settings.

CHAPTER 39

Loving Others

ARE YOU UNABLE TO LOVE OTHERS BECAUSE THE HURT THEY HAVE CAUSED you? *Arrividerci!* (Goodbye to it!) Give it up! I know from the cold, lonely, black-hole in my heart that will forever ache because I did not take five seconds to say three one-syllable words to my mother before her unforeseen yet instant death on a lonely stretch of highway.

I know it is not easy to give up anger, hurt or resentment. Italian *vendetta* is part of my genetic make-up, along with the *testadura*. But I realized that with each piece of emotional baggage I tossed overboard I have felt lighter. I picture the emotionally lighter me with less weight bearing upon arthritic joints. The same visualization can apply to the sore tissues of fibromyalgia,

or less weight for weak muscles and other neuromuscular illnesses, or less tugging at the heart strings for those with cardiac
problems.

Giving up the hurt you perceive has been caused by people,
God, the universe, or life frees you to love. But the freedom to
love starts by pulling on courage by the bootstraps and pitching
the heavy stockpile of stored hurts and resentment.

Have courage to:

- Say "*Arrividerci!*" to the feelings of hurt that hinder
  you from communicating your love to someone.

- Tell someone you love them, even if they have hurt
  you, or do not exhibit remorse or the desire to love
  you back.

- Remember to love yourself when you feel others do
  not love you.

CHAPTER 40
Love From Others

My cousin Stephen is an incredibly intelligent, deep-thinking, loving man. One evening we were gathered around my small kitchen table having a late night philosophical discussion. I was telling Stephen about how difficult it had been for me to ask other people to help me during the previous three months when, after an ankle fusion surgery, I had not been able to drive or bear weight on that leg.

"Lisa, you give love so much love to others, why can't you accept love from others? I have the same issue. I know I give love to other people but I have such a difficult time accepting love from someone else or love from the universe."

Stephen hit the nail head on. Of course I would take the day off from work and drive a friend an hour from Lansing to Ann Arbor if she needed a ride to her surgeon's office. Why then could I not bring myself to ask a friend if she would do the same for me after my ankle fusion surgeries? I could not step down on my foot and I was unable to maneuver into my car and safely drive in potential ice and snow. I kept telling myself what a burden it would be for someone to take their entire day; pick me up, put my wheelchair in the trunk, drive an hour, take the wheelchair out, wheel me into the surgeon's office, wait the two-plus hours for the cast to be sawed off and X-rays taken, doctor consultation and cast replaced. I created much angst tormenting myself about how I would get to and from the post-operative appointments.

In your time of need there are friends, neighbors, church members and relatives who desire to help and who desire to give you love. When I rejected acts of kindness out of the belief I was a burden, I was in effect denying those individuals that good feeling inside that I know I get from helping another.

My life is rich with countless acts of kindness from others such that I could fill a book.

I had had my second knee replacement a week before the anniversary of my mother's and grandmother's fatal auto accident The plan was to be discharged from the hospital before Christmas Day, but my red blood cell count was on a down-slide, and part of the surgical incision looked rebelliously non-adhering and infected. St. Joseph Hospital in North Hollywood, California was far from my sister, brothers and father back in Michigan. I was alone in my hospital room trying to deal with my thoughts about being hospitalized on Christmas Day and the impending first year anniversary of my mother's fatal car accident.

My friend Karen stuck her head into the door of my hospital room. "Are you decent?" she asked with a tinge of trouble-making fun in her voice. "Because I have some good-looking men here that want to see you."

Bounding in behind her were Karen's boyfriend Kerry and our mutual friend Tom. They were loaded with bags and an oddly wrapped Christmas present. Out from the bags came strings of Christmas lights and decorations that Karen brought from her home so as to cheer me. I was on the orthopedic ward. As with every orthopedic patient with surgical wounds to the lower extremities, my hospital bed had had a sturdy metal bar running lengthwise, four feet above me. Dropped down from the bar were chain links attached to a metal triangle-shaped hand grip for me to pull my body up while lying in bed. Karen had graduated from my alma mater, Mount Saint Mary's College's nursing school. She ordered the guys to wrap strings of lights around the bar above me. When the lights were plugged into the electrical outlet on the wall at the head of my bed, the room glowed … as did my spirits … and I felt loved!

Tom nervously shuffled closer to hand me the long and narrow present, wrapped in terribly crumpled Christmas paper. I had no idea what lay beneath the wrinkled uneven paper, but his gallant wrap effort brought its own joy to me. From the very first tear of wrapping paper I saw it was a fishing pole!

Tom, bless his heart, had bought me a Shakespeare fishing pole and casting reel. "This is so we can go fishing after you recover."

After Karen, Kerry and Tom left the nurse came into my room. She looked at the lights and said, "I am not sure Christmas lights are allowed on this floor, but I guess the question will have to wait until the day shift tomorrow." Her wink signaled to me no one was going to remove the lights from my room for awhile.

When it was time for "lights out" I asked the nurse to keep the Christmas lights plugged in. All alone that night I did not feel sorrow for spending the many Christmas Eve hours in the hospital without my mother, grandmother or Michigan family. Instead, I basked in the glow of the many twinkling, colored lights. I felt special and loved in a profound and fulfilled way. Karen, Kerry and Tom had brought me immeasurable joy and the most incredible gift of all: *amore.*

A second act of kindness example involved my friend Ruth. My mother had trained me in soprano harmony at a young age. Whenever I heard a melody, my brain automatically formulated a soprano descant. But this aptitude was not so with alto harmony. I usually needed to sight read the alto companion to a melody. All the more I admired and appreciated my friend Ruth for her alto talent.

While college students, Ruth and I planned the music to enhance the Biblical text that was part of each Sunday evening's student Mass held in the college chapel. As we grew deeper in the understanding of our Catholic faith through liturgy planning so did our friendship. We found enjoyment singing in choirs. Weekend evenings brought spontaneous song-fests with a small group of friends, Ruth leading us with her guitar. The pinnacle of our singing career and friendship was selection to sing the meditation song at our Baccalaureate Mass. There were four of us, including Ruth singing the alto and me singing soprano, singing "Come To Me" by Bob Hurd.

> *Come, come unto me. I will make you a jewel. Precious and rare, the glory you'll bear, in the crown of God.*

The song seemed to have been written for us as we sang from our souls the day before graduation.

After graduation the events of rheumatoid arthritis robbing my ability to walk, the tragic deaths of my mother and grandmother, and the onset of myasthenia gravis all converged into my needing placement in a nursing home. The culmination of all these events were a dark time in my life.

It was before the advent of cell phones and there was no phone in my nursing home room, so communication with friends was nearly impossible. Early one morning while I was in my hospital bed I lay awake but eyes were closed. The neglected breakfast tray lay across my lap. Unexpectedly, Ruth strolled into my room with guitar case in hand. How did she know my heart could use a good dose of singing?

"Come on," she said, "we need to get you out of bed. I thought we would provide music for the Sunday Mass here at the nursing home." She then swung my wheelchair close enough to the bed to lift me into it.

There was no calendar in my room but I knew it had to be the weekend because they had not taken me away early for the painful plasma pheresis procedure.

"I already cleared your room leave with the nurses; as long as I wheel you down to the chapel and bring you back it is okay," said Ruth, as she hurried me along. She wrapped a blanket over my shoulders in an effort to make my nursing home gown decent for Mass and plopped me into the wheelchair.

I put her music folder in my lap. Ruth configured a means to simultaneously balance the guitar case and push a wheelchair and we were off to the chapel.

Ruth explained to Father F. that we wanted to perform music during the Mass that morning. We searched for a sign of approval, but his face showed neither acquiescence nor disapproval. To this day, we have no idea what he thought of the impromptu arrangement. Undaunted, Ruth and I picked out some of our favorites songs, knowing our vocal arrangements would fall into place from the years of prior practice and performance. Father F. never looked over to us, rather, Ruth respectfully interrupted with guitar at the appropriate liturgical cues for song. There were a handful of people attending Mass and it would be televised into the rooms of patients who were unable to attend in person. I sat erect, as dignified as I could manage in my immodest hospital gown and blue plastic wheelchair.

I was overcome with gratitude for Ruth. Not only was I able to attend the Catholic Mass, I was also able to sing with my favorite alto. What I did not realize at the time, for just those few moments, I was not a nursing home patient, but rather, I was ministering to others through music.

With courage you can:

- Graciously ask for help from others.
- Express gratitude for acts of kindness bestowed on you.
- Bestow acts of kindness on others.

CHAPTER 41

Love From Others at the Time of Loss

I FOUND IT AGONIZINGLY DIFFICULT TO DEAL WITH THE GRIEF OF MY MOTHER'S and grandmother's sudden deaths. I have no magic formula to whisk away the intense heartache of grieving the ones you love. But I offer this suggestion from my own experience: in times of loss allow the love of others to heal and soothe you.

In the two-year period of time immediately preceding my mother's and grandmother's accident I was at times locked by pain into a fetal position. The joints in my elbows, hands and feet were so inflamed I could not use them to propel myself in the wheelchair. Instead, I would push myself slowly backward with my heels or grip the floor with my heels to move slowly forward around the tiny apartment. Because of the mobility limitations I was not able to propel over the raised door threshold to get outside. I had limited interaction with the world outside of the Woodland Hills, California apartment for those two years.

My mother and grandmother were the ones with whom I shared my day-to-day joys, concerns, stories, reflections and frustrations and with whom I exchanged hugs and human touch. They were my exclusive companions and my connection to the outer world. Although I had endured several tough health breaks for a person in her early twenties, I never could have imagined how ever-present the aching, lonely void of loss could be after their abrupt absence. Their familiar companionship and human touch were ripped away, never again to be experienced.

While lost in the cold dark void of grief, an instinct is to block feeling any future love while the sting of loss lingers. For me, the stabbing grief and gut-wrenching feeling of loss was soothed by being held long and closely by another being. Human touch was never more important for survival. It also helped me to talk about my grief, perhaps to have a person sit and listen while I told the same story of my mother or grandmother again and again, trying to make sense of what happened. For those who allowed me to cry without exhibiting their own discomfort at my display of emotion I can never thank them enough for allowing me to release raw, pent emotion in a safe environment without feeling shame, weakness or guilt.

I never would have expected how tremendously I missed the ability to share mundane comments such as, "Hey, the grocery store has bananas on sale this week". To sit alone in a room and realize the two people who would have listened with interest to my banana sale notification could no longer hear my voice, made my inner cry of anguish echo through the vast void in my heart.

The most significant human gestures which helped me survive devastating loss were those wrapped in the love of others. It took a lot of courage not to shrink away from feeling love. The self-preservation instinct at the time was to never allow love into my heart again. Without holding love for another meant I would never have to feel the anguish of loss. But it was the gentle little love packages from others which allowed me to love again.

With courage you can:

- Pamper yourself in the love from others at a time of grieving.
- Touch a lonely person's hand.
- Give a grieving person a close and long hug.
- Sit and be present with a person who is grieving.
- Be an active listener to someone who needs to express grief.
- Allow the selfless purpose of listening to wash away your uncomfortable feelings about witnessing tears, anger, sobs or hearing stories of a death experience.
- Love again after the loss of a loved one.

CHAPTER 42

The Importance of Giving Love to a Caregiver

THE JOB OF CAREGIVER IS OFTEN A THANKLESS JOB. A CAREGIVER CAN BE stretched beyond emotional and physical limits but the person receiving care may not be able to physically, mentally or emotionally express thanks.

Christmas 1985 was upon us. My sister Laura and I were living in Los Angeles with my mother and Hungarian grandmother. At the last minute, Laura and I decided to fly to Michigan to spend the Christmas holiday with Nonna, my father and two brothers. We landed a pretty good deal on airline tickets by using unpopular flight dates and times. Scoring affordable, rare, last-minute holiday seats was our sign that the trip was to be.

My mother drove us to LAX airport, masterfully maneuvering into a spot at the frantic crowded departure curb and popped the hatch on her white Gremlin. She and Laura got out, lifted the hatch, lifted out the luggage and somehow tugged and forced my wheelchair out from the tight Gremlin hatchback. Laura opened the now-freed, collapsed wheelchair, swung it close to the front passenger door and locked the brake on each large wheel.

The fact that Laura was traveling with me was a bonus. She was tall and strong, and she knew the proper way to transfer me from the car seat to the wheelchair. I could not make any steps on my own at this point due to the total arthritic destruction of knee joint cartilage. To transfer me from one seated location to another was mostly a dead-weight lift. Laura knew to grab me under my armpits, therefore reducing any pressure and damage to my inflamed elbow, wrist and hand joints. If an unknowing person tried to lift me by tugging on my hands or forearms, it would send my hands, wrists and elbows into a terrible flare-up.

Next was the perplexing question of how to get two suitcases, two carry-on bags, a wheelchair and a non-ambulatory sister to the airline check-in counter. Laura wedged a suitcase upright between my legs so that its narrow width end and its weight rested on the inner platform of my foot pedals. She piled the two bursting carry-on bags onto my lap, each jammed to a side of the upright suitcase. With brute strength born of necessity, she picked up her heavy suitcase with her stronger right hand and pushed me in the over-laden wheelchair with the other hand. It was not too far to the check-in counter even though we stopped several times before we made it to the counter to readjust shifting loads and for Laura to get a better grip or shove the wheelchair into a corrected course.

Absent the two pieces of monster luggage at check-in, I thought it would be an easier go. But, this was after all Los Angeles

International Airport. There were people of all shapes, sizes and colors; throngs of people in that pre-9/11 era where entire families accompanied a single family member for send-off. There were sprinters frantically dashing to reach a departure gate before their flights left; lollygag groups meandering, and spread four abreast across the walkway, totally oblivious or inconsiderate of the fact they were blocking the path for others; mothers pushing strollers; airplane crew members pulling rolling suitcases; and those airport passenger-carrying carts intended to courier passengers with ambulatory problems across the vast expanse of airport terminal, the cart's piercingly loud "beep, beep, beep, beep" parting the crowds in every direction. Through this chaotic mass of humanity and machinery Laura treacherously veered a person and bag-laden wheelchair through the long LAX traverse to our boarding gate.

Laura answered the call for pre-boarding and grasped the wheelchair hand grips as she pulled back hard against the force of the jet way's steep decline. At the airplane door she picked me up out of my wheelchair (the chair was too wide to fit into the airplane cabin) pivoted her body in a bear-hug with mine, and deposited me into the narrow, high-backed airplane aisle wheelchair. One of the airplane crew wheeled me backward to the first-row bulkhead seating, Laura following. At the row, Laura lifted me under my arms, pivoted, and deposited me in the aisle seat. Up, pivot, down. Laura had already employed the procedure several times for me that day but would have to employ the transfer procedure again after landing, waiting first for all passengers to deplane. Again, she would navigate and weave through the airport to collect our luggage and then transfer into our father's car.

Laura would get a reprieve when we pulled up into the driveway of Dad's modest red brick ranch. Our two brothers, both over six feet tall, both with bodies of athletes, came out the front door, sweatshirt, no coats (despite the frigid temperature) untied boots that had been pulled on hastily, and treaded through the four inches of snow to the car. My brother Paul picked me up as if nothing but a long, limp body pillow, and carried me through the snow, up the two cement steps and into the warm house. My other brother Peter grabbed the wheelchair and suitcases and brought them into the house.

As with many Italian families, we grew up spending time at holidays, weddings, summer vacations and assorted parties with our Italian *cugini* (cousins.) Laura and I were the only cousins who lived outside of Michigan. So as our visit was an event meriting respect, it called for a gathering of Dad's first cousins. He answered the door and took Great-Aunt Victoria, Nonna's sister, by the arm to help her into the back room where Nonna, Laura and I awaited the arrival of *cugini*. Great-Aunt Victoria stopped at Nonna for a *baci* (kiss). Following her was Great-Aunt Victoria's daughters and son-in-law, Aunt Fran, Uncle Carl and Aunt Jo.

Everyone gathered around me. Hugs and kisses were exchanged between questions about how I was feeling, how my flight went, and explaining to which saint they were praying for intercession with God for my healing. Laura had moved her way forward for hugs and kisses, but was again neglected in the background.

After a period of time, a loud question cut through the conversation that had encircled me. "What about me?" It was Laura's voice, but it sounded much younger than her 22 years. "Doesn't anyone care about me?" There was hurt and some anger in her tone.

Laura was absolutely right. She had exerted a tremendous amount of time and energy to get me to this gathering in Michigan. She, too, had experienced a range of emotions as she provided care for me the past year. It was important for me, as the person struggling with a fierce disease to receive and feel the love and support of family. But it was also important for Laura to receive and feel love and support as well.

As often occurs, a visitor inquires about the person with a serious illness, but no inquiry is made about the caregiver. The person with the serious illness is struggling physically and emotionally, but the caregiver is often struggling with emotion and physical fatigue as well. Yet the caregiver's wellbeing is often overlooked. That Laura cared for me out of *amore* is indisputable. That I felt a tremendous amount of *amore* and gratitude toward Laura for all the care she gave me is indisputable. But I cannot remember having told her how appreciative I was for all she had done to get me to Michigan to be surrounded by loving family. I am also ashamed to think of the hundreds of family, friends and strangers to whom I have not adequately expressed my appreciation. I know I would not be where I am today without that good care and love, nor do I know how to impress upon them adequately what that care and love has meant to me.

In addition to the phenomenon of overlooking caregivers there is the paradox of the patient appearing to be unappreciative, demanding or frustrated with the caregiver. Remember the carrot juice gulping story? It was my feelings of loss of control over my body that led me to be controlling and demanding of my selflessly caring mother. My message to a patient: before becoming frustrated or before having hurt feelings put yourself into the shoes of the caregiver. Try to be as objective as possible and try to see the perspective from their position. My message to a caregiver: before becoming frustrated or having hurt feelings put yourself into the shoes of the patient. Try to be as objective as possible and try to see the perspective from their position.

During the Catholic Liturgy there is a segment where the congregation as a whole offers prayers of intention for identified issues or people. At my parish, there is always a general prayer intention: "For those who are sick and *for those who care for them.*" That last phrase should not go unnoticed. The volunteers at my church understand that the caregiver needs support just as much as the person who is ill. Hospice gets it right by paying attention to the caregiver while the patient is alive and by not abandoning the caregiver after a loved one's death. Hospice understands that a physically and emotionally supported caregiver is better able to serve her loved one, and after the passing of a loved one, the caregiver may be emotionally and physically depleted. The best nourishment for the depletion? *Amore. Moltissimo amore.* (Very much love). Or *grande amore* (big love) to use a phrase I adore.

You may not even recognize you are a caregiver or the vital impact you make in someone's life.

Debbie Kershinik came from a family of practicing women nurses. Her mother was a nurse. Debbie graduated in my class with a Bachelor of Nursing degree. Debbie's sister, Mary, graduated the year after us with a Bachelor of Nursing degree. Mrs. Kershisnik, Debbie and Mary were graced with sweet, happy and generous dispositions. They also stood out for their physical beauty: tall, slim, with broad, white ever-present smiles. Mrs. Kershisnik became one of my surrogate moms after my mother died; she enveloped me in her sweet care and love.

Debbie and I lived on the third floor of the Carondelet dormitory at Mount St. Mary's College. Debbie's roommate, Donna, was a physical therapy major.

Donna had warned me before my first knee replacement surgery, "It is really going to hurt after surgery."

I have serious pain every day of my life. How worse can the surgical pain be?

I went by myself to the hospital the morning of the surgery. The wheelchair transport van arrived about 5:00 a.m.; the sun had not yet illumined the cold October night's darkness. The van driver loaded me in my wheelchair, strapped down the wheelchair for security and drove from my apartment in the San Fernando Valley to the North Hollywood hospital. I knew that I would have no family or friends waiting during or after surgery and I was okay with that. My sister had moved and the surviving members of my family were all in Michigan. Why should a friend take a day from work to sit in a hospital while I was not even conscious?

I waited in pre-op alone and the surgery was performed without a loved one present. I felt myself pulling out of the darkness of anesthesia and into consciousness. My eyes fluttered open to bright light. Then it hit. *Pain!* Pain slammed against the surgical site with such forceful intensity my whole being clenched in a grimace. Then darkness resumed as I plunged back into unconscious. It was if the sensory portion of my brain saw the tidal wave of incoming pain sensation that was about to come crashing over it and shut itself down.

Bright, dazzling light again. This time the light stayed long enough for me to hear the beeping of medical machinery around me. The heavy force of pounding pain rushed in. *You must be in the recovery room.* I tried to focus my open eyes but the fluorescent lights on the ceiling directly above my face seemed extraordinarily bright. Suddenly an angel appeared before my eyes. The angel's face blocked the harshness of the artificial light but had a radiance of its own. She was the most beautiful angel with blond hair, blue eyes, and large white smile to match her white garments. "Lisa." Her voice was so sweet and soothing to my aching senses. "Lisa?" This time the soft voice spoke my name as if asking. I tried to gather as much sense as possible to focus better on my angel.

"Lisa, it's Mom Kershisnik. I was able to switch schedules with a coworker so I could be your recovery room nurse. Your surgery is over, honey."

I struggled to keep my eyes open and focused on the angelic form.

"Lisa, it's Mom Kershisnik. Your surgery went really well. Everything is okay, honey."

Mom Kershisnik? Yes, I could see more clearly now. My angel *was* Mrs. Kershinik. The radiance was from her beautiful smile. The white garments were her nurse uniform. I tried to utter a word but my throat felt dry from the anesthesia and hurt from the intubation tube, and my throat had swelled from emotion. No matter what age or level of maturity, every person needs a mother to remind her "everything is alright" at the moment of life's most desperate situations where fear is replaced by assurance. That is *amore*. A mother's love is powerful.

My biological mother had died months earlier. I came to the hospital alone with the expectation that I would be without family on the day of surgery and the belief that everything would be fine. Mrs. Kershinik had indeed swapped schedules so she could be a recovery room nurse the day and time of my surgery. She had not wanted to give me false hope and then not be able to work the recovery room and thus I did not have the expectation of seeing her. I had never had a major surgery without a family member present. Mrs. Kershisnik's presence had an enormously significant impact on my emotional wellbeing and physical healing. She did not have to go out of her way to be in the recovery room that day. To this day I wonder if she knows that her being at my recovery room bedside was a significant part of my emotional support for that knee replacement recovery.

There are so many who have imparted love and care for me in ways they believe were insignificant, but for which I count as part of my riches today. Inside my treasure chest of riches is *molto amore*.

To Mom Roberge and Mom Richman: you called me "Darling" and "My Love." To every mother who gathered this motherless daughter into their embrace, I lapped up every bit of your affection and basked in your motherly love. *"Tanti grazie per sua amore."* (Thank you very much for your love.)

For the countless family and friends who have pushed me in my wheelchair, gone shopping for me, brought me food, driven me to doctor appointments, made me smile, and prayed for me:

"Tanti grazie per sua amore." (Thank you very much for your love.)

With courage you can:

- View a situation from your caregiver's perspective instead of from your expectation.

- Do an honest review of an incident, including a caregiver's position, before adopting hurt feelings or a frustrated attitude.

- Always express gratitude to a caregiver despite whether the care met your expectations.

CHAPTER 43

That's Amore. Dating When You Look Disabled or "Different"

"When the moon hits your eye like a big-a pizza pie ... That's amore!"

That's Amore, the tune Dean Martin and Jerry Lewis made legendary from their slapstick scene in the 1953 movie, *The Caddy.* My mother and I had our own comedic duet version we performed at parties. Mom was the straight-guy, Dean Martin-melody and I the funny sidekick on parody echo and harmony. We had performed it so many times for others or ourselves that we could splendidly pull it off right on the spot with no practice or forewarning. And we always managed a laugh, if not too much chuckle from the audience at least a laugh at ourselves.

The famous lead chorus line, "*When the moon hits your eye like a big-a pizza pie … That's amore!*" spoofs Italian-Americans in its seeming unromantic image. But to me, as an Italian-American, it speaks truth. Aspects of love can be brutal and feel like being hit straight in the face with a hot, greasy slab of dough. Aspects of love and intimacy can be especially brutal if you are a person who looks or acts "different" than society has defined as "normal".

One Friday morning, May 20, 2005, I heard the voice of a Vicky Page, a 26-year-old woman from New York Story Corps: Recording America on National Public Radio's Morning Edition, recording her story, "Learning to Live with Cerebral Palsy".

> *As far as intimate relationships, being in a wheelchair you are always protected by this chair. There is always armor between you and the opposite sex. So intimacy is a difficult thing. You know, I've never been kissed. So I have no idea what the norms are of a relationship.*

I could relate to the sadness in her voice as she poignantly told of her struggle to experience intimacy while seated in a wheelchair.

Before being diagnosed with rheumatoid arthritis, down-hill skiing was a passion of mine. Downhill snow-skiing is a great Michigan winter sport. The year after I graduated from law school I went with a group of friends for a weekend ski trip. We stayed at a friend's family ski chalet in the Northwest portion of the state. I was not able to ski but I had brought work up to the ski resort; I was content to gain ground on my contentious litigation cases while my friends skied during the day. In the evenings, we visited one of the small town bars, packed with down-state yuppies.

"Hi … want to dance?" asked the quite handsome, visibly muscular guy.

I was not sure how to explain that I had rheumatoid arthritis in the awkward moment between someone catching your eye and going for it. I glanced toward what was a makeshift dance floor and realized that it was a corner of the bar, bordered by tall bar tables, and it was packed.

Mark and I danced the rest of the night, if you could call it that. The makeshift dance floor was so tightly jammed that we mostly bobbed up and down, no room for swinging arms or twirling. It was the perfect scenario for a dancer with artificial knees, and corroded ankle and shoulder joints. It was amazing the amount of info we exchanged despite the blaring DJ tunes.

Mark was from a Detroit suburb close to Lansing. We talked for hours the following week and he asked me to meet for dinner the following Saturday. He said he was thrilled to meet an intelligent female attorney. "I can hardly believe I met you. You are the best thing since sliced bread."

Such a corny cliché, I thought, but oh how wonderful it sounded coming from this man.

Mark was an engineer with one of the big three auto companies. He was smart, had a steady and well-paying job and appeared he took good care of his health.

I arrived at our meeting place where Mark greeted me with a huge smile and a strong hug. He helped me off with my 80s style winter puffy, down coat and I followed him in the direction that he motioned. But then I stopped dead in my tracks.

"Why are you walking like that?" His tone was not kind.

"What do you mean?"

"You are hunched and limping," he said unsympathetically and accusatorily.

What is going on? Surely he had noticed last Saturday that I had rheumatoid arthritis. Come to think of it, we had found so much in common to discuss I could not recall the subject coming up despite the hours we had spent on the phone.

"I have rheumatoid arthritis. You knew that."

"I did not know that." His voice was mean.

"We danced for hours, surely you noticed?"

"No, obviously I did not notice," followed by an incredibly uncomfortable silence.

"Why didn't you tell me about it this week?" again, in an accusatory tone.

"Cuz … as I explained before, I thought you had noticed over the four hours we spent together dancing," I replied nervously.

"Cuz? Cuz? What kind of lawyer are you going to be if you use a non-word such as "cuz?" He was in full critical mode, acting out his anger.

What had I done to provoke such negative attitude and anger? *This is not really happening.* My dream evening was quickly turning into my worst nightmare. My stomach felt twisted and the meal was brief. I made a gesture to leave and he directly ushered me out without even allowing me the opportunity to put on my coat before entering the frigid winter evening.

The experience shook my being to the extent I did not date again for a long time. I knew better intellectually yet it was very hard not let it diminish my belief in myself as a good person. The importance of a solid self-love was never more important. I felt as though no one could love me because my disabilities were a turn-off and a burden

I never wanted to be married before thirty years old. I wanted to put all my focus into becoming a doctor, specializing in surgery and doing missionary work. I always thought that when I finished the preparatory portion of my life-calling, my soul mate would appear and life would be happy ever after. As I approached my late thirties and I was not married, I confided in a friend that I wanted to meet my "someone special."

As she started going through the list of her and her husband's single male friends, she stopped suddenly and remarked, "That's right, you need someone special, a person who can deal with disabilities."

Her statement was startling. I realized she thought of my disabilities as liabilities. But I saw it differently. The presence of disabilities had forged a resilient emotional fortitude; better to see up front an individual's physical disability characteristics than discover after marriage the non-disabled spouse's non-visible, deeply-rooted emotional disabilities. Plus, there is no guarantee that death or disability may surprise the non-disabled person tomorrow no matter how young or how much money one possess.

Thankfully, I have had more fun and affirming dating experiences than negative ones. The most important lesson for me in all of the good and bad experiences is being strong in your self-love is the optimal way to loving others and to attracting an emotionally healthy and loving mate.

With courage you can:
- See yourself for the special person you are.
- Love yourself for the special person you are.
- Love again, even if you have been hurt by love.

CHAPTER 44

The Marriage Relationship and Chronic Illness

It was a huge disappointment in Nonna's life that I did not marry and have children before turning 40 years old, nor did she hide that sentiment from me. She expressed it in true Italian passive-aggressive fashion when I was in my thirties and then quite blatantly at the threshold of 40.

There is a favorite story told by my brother Paul. Paul is an attorney who started his own law practice which includes a small portion of estate law, wills and trusts. The estate law clientele, in Italian-American fashion, includes many family, friends, and friends of family.

An infamous story involves one such Italian family friend. At Nonna's request Paul respectfully agreed to assist elderly Emily with her will and estate planning. As Emily often desired changes to her will, Paul had several occasions to speak one-on-one with her.

On one such occasion Emily gushed, "Paul, your grandmother is so proud of you. She always is heard boasting to others, 'Oh Paul, he is a lawyer!'"

Paul graciously accepted the compliment.

Then unexpectedly Emily launched into, "But isn't it too bad about Lisa?"

Paul had no idea what Emily was talking about and did not respond.

"You know, your grandmother and I talk about poor Lisa; she's not married. We pray to Fr. Solanus to find her a husband."

Paul did all he could not to emit a loud laugh and as soon as he finished his conversation with Emily he called me.

When I picked up the receiver I heard his deep, extended laughter. "Now I know what Nonna and her friends really think about the two of us," he exclaimed.

We both got a kick out of the fact that it did not matter that I had overcome two serious illnesses, made it through law school, litigated precedent-setting cases fresh from law school and at that time was policy advisor to the Michigan Senate. None of these remarkable accomplishments seemed to matter. I was not a success because I was not married and with children.

There are advantages and disadvantages to being a single person with a disability. My friend Fay was diagnosed with myasthenia gravis shortly after the birth of her daughter. Fay was beautiful and glamorous, her husband a strikingly handsome, successful international businessman. Before her diagnosis, they enjoyed a very active life together in California's San Fernando Valley.

Fay had a difficult case of myasthenia gravis. Often before noon time she had lost the muscle strength to speak and the muscles in her legs became too weak to walk after short distances. She stopped accompanying her husband on business trips overseas and often cancelled their evening social events, being overcome by fatigue by 5:00 p.m.

Fay believes her marriage survived the changes a serious illness brings because she and her husband openly discussed each other's feelings about the changes. Compromises were made by both spouses, and they tried not to blame or punish.

Fay explained that it was more difficult dealing with chronic autoimmune diseases when you were married because you feel the guilt of holding your spouse back or that you are a burden on them. I responded that it would be easier if married because you would have a spouse to help open a bottle of medication, carry in the heavy grocery sacks, and drop you off at the entrance of the shopping center—all the day-to-day events that cause deterioration of the joints or muscle weakness. Being single also carried the worry of being a sole provider of economic income or health insurance benefits.

On what did Fay and I agree? That single versus married, when it comes to having a chronic disability, is similar to the age-old "the grass is greener on your side of the fence" debate.

With courage it is possible to:

- Have your marriage survive by openly discussing in respectful, gentle, caring terms, feelings about your own or a spouse's illness.
- Avoid destructive blame, guilt and punishment.
- Make compromises in the marriage relationship for the changes an illness may bring.

CHAPTER 45

Remembering to Love Yourself When Others are not Loving Toward You

"DON'T LET THE BAD GUYS GET YOU DOWN." I HAVE REPEATED THIS PHRASE to myself and friends over and over again. I believe in it more as proverb than cliché. Its premise is essential for maintaining self-love and keeping hope alive. When I have not heeded this statement I have slipped into self-doubt and self-criticism, essentially straying from loving myself.

The "bad guy" may not be the proverbial evil figure seated on a horse with black cowboy hat and razor-sharp spurs. That bad guy may be your family member, friend or spouse, perhaps acting with intent or with ignorance, making it all the more important to possess a healthy sense of respect for yourself.

I had finally made the decision to attend law school. My brother Paul, already attending the University of Detroit School of Law, talked me through endless questions and concerns. I had prayed fervently about the decision. I had also conferred with my rheumatologist, Dr. Laing and Associate Dean Maveal at University of Detroit School of Law. Decision-making had been a tedious experience, but I had finally reached a peacefulness and excitement about the decision.

I called a college friend to share the news that I would soon be entering law school. She was a brilliant, bubbly woman, one of the few pre-med classmates who actually made it into medical school. She had been a lifesaver after my mother and grandmother had been killed, and leaving me without family in California, would call me from Michigan several times a week. She knew more than most people the depth of my heartbreak about not being able to attend medical school.

I called her in the middle of her day and blurted my happy news about going to law school.

"You *can't* go to law school!" Her voice was darkly condemnatory.

It was not the response I had expected. The air had been sucked from my lungs and I was physically unable to respond.

"What do you think you are doing?" came the next round of attack. "First you are getting a Master's Degree in counseling. Then you are going to be a hospital chaplain. Now you are going to try law school? You can't keep changing your mind! This is the most absurd thing I every heard!" she chided in a stern, critical tone.

When I hung up the phone I was spinning with self-doubt and self-condemnation. I remember clearly sitting on the edge of Nonna's bed, hand still gripping the brown plastic handset of her 70s style square phone, staring blankly at the lavender, quilted, polyester bedspread. I felt sick with upheaval. With dragging feet and bowed head I walked into Nonna's front room.

Nonna looked up from the novel she was reading from her reclined position on the couch. "Leeza, honey, what happened?"

I slumped in the open space on the couch left by her short legs and started mindlessly caressing her toes, all the time telling her about the surprising conversation.

"*Leeza*, do not pay attention to those people who make you feel bad. *Coraggio, Leeza*! Listen to what your brother Paul told you. He encouraged you. Follow your heart, *Leeza*." She spoke with emphatic hand gestures.

The telephone conversation was an important lesson, though easy to tell now, was tormenting and drawn out at the time. All of Paul's encouragement and Nonna's heart-felt, hand-emphasized support were at risk of being extinguished. My so called friend's forceful reproach had really shaken me. I actually thought about not going to law school, telling myself that if such a good friend had had such a reproachful response to my attending law school, maybe it was not the best idea. The time I spent working through the negative feelings about myself and my law school plans was time I should have been spending preparing for the quickly approaching first term.

I think back on how I gave serious consideration to not attending law school based on this woman's strong opinion. If I had not gone to law school I would not have helped all the people with disabilities, myself being a disability rights attorney. If I had not gone to law school I would not have had the opportunity to work on vital state and federal social policy as a state senate policy advisor and a governor's policy coordinator, and make significant decisions as an administrative law judge. I might never have had a self-supporting job with good health insurance, integral to managing life with physical limitations. The Jimmy Stewart *It's a Wonderful Life* phenomenon.

Don't let the bad guys get you down! Coraggio!

All the expanding rings of good potential were forgone because of the comments of a friend. It was a tough lesson on possessing a fortress of self-respect strong enough to withstand a sneak attack by friend instead of foe.

I have also received a staggering blow to my ego at times when I felt the most confident. I had gone to an Italian-American wedding shower shortly after taking the grueling Michigan state Bar examination. I was stuck in the awful three months limbo between taking the examination and being informed that I had passed it. I had been beating on prospective employers' doors, but with no success, the endeavor all the more difficult during the limbo's lack of Bar license. A wedding or bridal shower in my Italian-American family meant every relative extending back several times removed, and anyone you had ever met in your life with whom you had more than a two minute conversation was invited. Until I attended my college classmates' showers, I did not realize that bridal and wedding showers could have fewer than 200 participants and could be held in a location other than a local Knights of Columbus hall.

An Italian cousin of my father's had heard me telling another cousin that I was pursuing a career in patent law. She said that her husband had a friend who worked in a law firm and she thought he did some patent work. But it was not just any lawyer; it was a *senior partner* in a big firm that did a large proportion of patent law cases in the Detroit area. The husband of the Italian cousin called to tell me the senior partner would meet with me and to call his secretary to make an appointment. *Hallelujah!* This could be *mia buona fortuna!* (My good fortune)

As a new law school graduate my income was meager and my monthly law school loan payment hefty. My professional wardrobe consisted of a couple of dresses and a suit from a second-hand store. I also had an "interview suit," compliments of a generous friend who had given me a birthday gift certificate to Hudson's Department Store. The "How to Interview for a Legal Job" guides all said to wear a navy or black suit. I settled on the navy suit—double-breasted and boxy jacket with matching skirt that fell below the knee—the essence of propriety.

As I drove out to the meeting with the senior partner I felt good about the choice I had made in my attire. I had paired the suit with a high-collared white shirt, a fortunate second-hand store find, now highly pressed for the occasion; I had cut my hair short several months before. I felt ready to meet another professional, this one a senior partner at one of the top patent law firms in the Detroit area.

The distant relative clarified that the meeting was only to give me advice on finding an attorney position. But I couldn't help but have hopeful thoughts. Maybe there was a chance the senior partner was looking for a new associate to do some of the patent law grunt work. After all, I had a Bachelor's degree in science, a passion for biomedical issues and I was an extremely hard worker.

I even forgot about the fact that I looked like I had a disability and that I had a gap in work experience. I assured myself that as a senior partner in a law firm he knew the new body of disability rights law and would not directly ask about my arthritis or myasthenia gravis.

I pulled the heavy thick glass door, gold-emblazoned with names of the law firm's founding partners. The forceful resistance of the door won over my disease-worn elbows and the joints cracked in defeat. I froze my smile so as to not wince from the sharp, cracking elbow pain.

As I was directed to the senior partner's office, I noticed the trendy attired staff and caught a glimpse of one in uncomfortable appearing high-heeled shoes. I had not worn a heel higher than one inch since the year after I was diagnosed with rheumatoid arthritis. I was immediately self-conscious and fought not to look at my low heeled, thick rubber-soled pumps. *Do not pay any attention. You are here as a serious and potential lawyer.*

I entered an elaborate office and was greeted by a perfectly coifed, handsome man in his mid-fifties. We talked about the practice of patent law in general terms for about ten minutes. I brought up the topic of emerging trends in biotechnology. I incorporated into the conversation my passion for science and the fact that I possessed up-to-date knowledge of the cutting edge scientific and biotechnological advances. I felt good about imparting another reason why I would be an asset to his firm. I took a deep breath behind my smile. *The meeting is going well.* I then asked the senior partner about his experience with the firm. He verified the infamous pressure on law firm attorneys to accrue billable client hours.

It was quiet for a moment. He then asked about my disability, adding the question about how disability would affect my ability to work. As if the fact that he was asking was not shocking enough, the flat-out, non-apologetically, business manner added horror.

What? He can't ask about my disability.

The Americans with Disabilities Act had been signed into law a couple of years prior. Prospective employers were prohibited from asking potential employees about the employee's disability and how the disability would affect their work.

The smile that had prevailed on my face froze. Every bit of me did not want to discuss my disabilities. But how could I not answer? He was sitting across from me, staring at my face, waiting for me to respond. I gave a general response about having arthritis but kept it positive. I was glad I had practiced responses so I could at least stammer a rehearsed piece.

He stood and communicated through body language that the meeting was over. *Thank heavens.* I was desperate to be out of the hot seat.

He moved quickly before me so that I was still rising as he towered before me. I finished standing and he held out his hand to shake good-bye. I extended my hand, embarrassed at my crooked fingers. He grasped my hand and clamped down hard. *Ouch!* The arthritic bones in my fragile hand crunched. While still hand in hand, I uttered my gratitude and closing platitude.

He responded that it was "his pleasure" but hesitated as if thinking what to say next. "Maybe one of those women's organizations can take pity on you and help you." He offered the advice as if it were a gift from a sage.

Pity? I was appalled.

I did not need pity! I am sure my face turned red. I know there was a lump in my throat.

Now it was my turn to move quickly. With great haste I retreated from the affluent office. My hand was throbbing from the insensitive, hurtful handshake. It was moments after I had told him I had arthritis and yet he had forcefully crushed my delicate hand. My ego was totally deflated. Now I knew exactly what he thought about me. I was nothing more than a person who needed pity. This was a courtesy meeting of precious billable minutes donated out of a sense of pity.

I retraced my steps past the perfectly outfitted secretaries and felt woefully unsophisticated in my outdated, androgynous, orthopedic outfit. I slid quickly into a low self-worth pit. *Why did you think anyone would hire you?*

It was before cell phones were available and I was about a half hour from Nonna and my brother Paul.

By the time I reached Paul I could barely tolerate the lashings of worthlessness I had inflicted upon myself. I poured out an unstoppable story through anguished sobs, concluding with self-deprecating commentary. Paul waited a moment to make sure I had finished my purge, then started laughing.

"I told you so," was his lead-in comment. But I did not feel as if I was being chided. I instantly felt better because I knew where he was going.

"Why would you ever want to work in a law firm where people are insensitive and all focus is on earning billable hours to appease the firm's partners? You know your heart and soul, Lisa. You want to help people in the health care area. You can do so much to help improve health care for thousands of people with your law degree."

Paul was on one of his soapboxes, but by the time he stepped down I was refocused on recognizing my talents and life-fulfilling quests.

Every person should be so fortunate to have a brother like Paul. His strength and wisdom has several times pulled me from my own injurious thoughts and set me on the right course of belief in myself, hope and encouragement; not that I did not get a scolding from him for setting myself up in the patent law meeting situation to negative experiences and easily falling prey to my self-doubt.

Don't let the bad guys get you down! Coraggio!

Have the courage to:

- Not let the bad guys get you down!
- Reject the negative comments of others.
- Follow the stirrings of your heart despite what others tell you.
- Believe in the good you possess despite the judgment of others.

CHAPTER 46

The Courage to Love Yourself

Life may hand you *limoni* (lemons) the *Napolitano* (Naples) size of softballs. It is how you deal with those lemons that make a difference in the outcome for your life. You can believe you have the ability to make the proverbial successful lemonade or you can make the sour face.

In April 2008, I had finished the first draft of all four *Coraggio* books. Neck and shoulder X-rays were nonchalantly taken so my rheumatologist could track the cause of neck and right shoulder pain. Two days later I got a call from an orthopedic surgeon's office urgently requesting me to see the surgeon within the week.

The day before seeing the neck surgeon, without warning, intolerable pain struck both ankles. The pain was inhumanely malicious, stopping me mid-step and brutally assaulting any attempts to sleep at night. Because of the sudden onset and extreme degree of pain I thought the screws and plates in my ankles had come loose.

On an emergency basis I saw a new ankle surgeon. When he entered the exam room he blurted, "The good news is your ankle hardware is not loose. The bad news is that some of the bone tissue in your ankles is necrotic. That means part of your ankle bones are dead. My recommendation is amputation of both from the knee down. You'll thank me when I'm done."

With great effort I limped from the ankle surgeon's office to the neck surgeon's office. Merely hours after hearing the shocking ankle amputation recommendation, I listened to the neck surgeon say, "Several of the vertebrae in your neck have shifted out of place due to arthritic changes. Your spinal cord is being pinched. You need surgery as soon as possible because you could become paralyzed or die if your spinal cord is severed. I will cut though the front part of your neck and fuse your vertebrae with a metal plate. I will then place you in a halo brace after the surgery. The metal halo will be held in place with four screws inserted in your skull. You will wear the halo for at least three months. For most of the three months you will need someone to help you wash and dress."

The combination of dire prognoses was an incredible blow to absorb in a short period of time. Unexpectedly and within a two week time span, one surgeon had informed me my best option was double leg amputation, and a second surgeon had told me it was critical he fuse my neck and secure it with a heavy halo brace screwed into my skull for three months.

For the first time in a long time I cried. Every principle I had painstakingly laid out in the four *Coraggio* books was put to the test. I couldn't figure out how I could make it through those surgeries without burdening someone else. I hadn't cried over the prior seven major surgeries. *What is the difference now? Where is courage, my usual sidekick?*

I couldn't find courage to face the surgeries because I had lost it along with the ability to love myself. A few weeks earlier I had interpreted a person's callous comments toward me as negative. More unfortunately, I had *accepted* that person's words. With the acceptance of a negative view I had discarded love for me.

It took raw courage for me to shuck the negative view and believe in myself again. With the return of self-love, self-worth fell into place. *Occhi aprono!* (Eyes open!) With the return of self-love my eyes and mind were opened to the steps I needed to successfully leap over the onerous hurdles.

With courage came the strength to implement the steps forward. I prayed for the right surgeons and for the right solutions.

One year to the day of my fervent prayers my prayers had been answered. I had found a kind and courageous surgeon, Dr. Paul Fortin. I had begged him to believe in me, that I would do whatever needed to be done to replace the necrotic ankle bone tissue and I pleaded for a solution other than amputation. He believed in me and he agreed to replace the necrotic tissue with a newly available artificial ankle, a prosthesis more friendly to a rheumatoid arthritic ankle.

The developer of the Salto-Talaris prosthesis flew into Michigan and assisted Dr. Fortin with placement of my first artificial ankle prosthesis. It was a phenomenal success. In April 2009, one year after the amputation recommendation, I could walk again on my own two feet and without the heavy, sweaty, ugly black leather ankle braces.

I recalled that nursing home night when Nonna's words saved my life. I had no family in California; no spouse; no job. I hadn't been able to take one step in the prior two years. At the one year mark from that nursing home night I took my first steps. Since then I always had a roof over my head and food to eat. A new mantra was formed: *You are testadura. One year from now your situation will be different and all will be okay. You never have and never will go without food and shelter. For now, only focus on one minute at a time...one day at a time.*

One year from the devastating accident that took the lives of my mother and grandmother I took my first steps in years. One year from the devastating news that I needed an emergency neck fusion and my ankles needed to be amputated I took my first steps without the heavy black leather ankle braces. With the courage to love myself came the genuine inner-belief that no matter what devastation is thrown in my path, I will survive and I will once again laugh and sing.

I see Nonna in my mind as plain as if she were before me. Her jaw is set in that tight, determined *testadura* stance. She rejects the role of victim. She has the self-respect and self-love to recognize she is the one who is responsible for the outcome of her situation. It does not matter to her that she has a small stature, that her physical body is shrunken and weak, that she has the income of a widow's meager pension. She believes in the power of *coraggio* and she summons that *coraggio* to move forward with determination.

With this *coraggio* power Nonna forged *Lezione Tre: Amore* (Life Lesson Three: The Courage to Love), which taught me to have the courage to love myself when I felt unlovable, the courage to accept love from others, the courage to love despite being hurt, and the courage to love again after losing someone I dearly loved.

In 1921, Nonna set out on a trip that would take her to a land with unknown terror but hoped-for promise. As her tiny body bobbled along with the jostling cart, she watched the cactus dotting the arid landscape of Southern Italy. Cactus after cactus encroaching the dusty road that led her to a new life. From afar she thought the cactus plants were beautiful for their uniqueness;

some were tall and slender, others shorter and widespread. As the wagon passed close specimens she felt sorry for the plants misshapen by missing limbs or gnarled scars. From close proximity she could count the *fico d'India* (prickly pear) on each cactus. The bulbous, reddened, Italian prickly pear's shaped appeared funny and made her giggle. It reminded her of the rosacea-ruddied nose of the *streganonna* witch she heard in stories told by her grandmother ... bumps and whiskers included. One cactus passed closely enough for her to reach and pluck the fruit; her outreached hand stopped short out of fear for the sting of the protruding long black needles.

The prickly pear cactus symbolizes the brave, stubborn disposition of my Italian ancestors. It has a tough life as a plant, having to take hold in dry, poor and rocky soil, never knowing when or if it might receive a few life-sustaining drops of moisture. Nonetheless, its clings courageously to the soil upon which it rests, protecting itself from predators by many long, painful spines.

As my ancestors discovered, just beneath the stinging-barbed skin lay delicious, succulent, flesh, vibrant and nourishing. This ugly fruit provided the hydration and sustenance of many a traveling ancestor attempting the trek through hot, dry plains and mountains in an attempt to reach a neighboring town to trade goods.

I can relate to the missing-limbed, misshapen cactus. I have deeply gnarled scars from nine major surgeries and I admit I have mechanisms similar to spiny pickers for preventing a person's love from coming too close.

"*Coraggio, Leeza. Coraggio.*"

I think of Nonna words of encouragement and I am reminded to use courage to peel back the skin of my prickly pear. It is only by courage that I can see directly below the appearance surface how special I truly am. With courage I recognize that I possess the love and willingness to be vibrant and nourishing to others.

It takes courage to believe in yourself and love who you are. With Nonna's example, I recognized from a young age how precious is each day of my life and to appreciate each day despite illness or pain. I experienced how easily a life and a loved one can vanish and set out to cherish my loved ones despite resentment or hurts.

By beginning with loving myself I have been able to treasure and enjoy the interactions of each day. And on the days I live with *amore* worries about my disabilities and loss seem few, and chronic joint pains feel subdued. With the energy freed from worry and stamina freed from pain, I create a day of "I can!" while shouting *"Coraggio!"* while singing *"Amore!"* and while radiating hope and joy to those I meet.

With courage you can:

- Love yourself.
- Operate from an inner core of self-love.
- Spread to others the hope, joy and positive energy that emanates from your inner core of self-love.
- Live with *amore* so worries about illness and loss seem few and chronic joint pain feels subdued.

Epilogue

More *Coraggio* coming soon! Nonna was merely getting started in her *Lezioni Uno-Tre*.

Coraggio! Lessons for Living from an Italian Grandmother: Courage to Believe in Miracles

> *Lezione Quattro* (Lesson Four): The courage to believe in faith, hope, prayers, healing and miracles. Expected Fall 2010

Coraggio! Lessons for Living from an Italian Grandmother: Courage to Conquer Pain

> *Lezione Cinque* (Lesson Five): The courage to discover new perspectives and approaches to dealing with physical and emotional pain. Expected Fall 2011

Epilogue

Coraggio! Lessons for Living from an Italian Grandmother: The Courage to Grieve and to Honor (bring peace, love and joy to) the End of Life

Lezioni Sei & Sette (Lessons Six & Seven): The courage to honor the end-of-life and live each day as if you are creating your legacy. Expected Spring 2011

www.withcourageican.com

Bibliography

2005 Dietary Guidelines Advisory Committee Report, issued January 2005.

Alden, Doug. *Utah Study Links Obesity and Bad Knees.* May 6, 2005, Associated Press.

Arthritis Foundation (800 283-7800), www.arthritis.org

Cousins, Norman. *The Anatomy of an Illness as Perceived by the Patient: Reflections on Healing and Regeneration.* 1979. Bantam Books, New York. pp. 28-45, 82-87.

Goode, Erica. *Can an Essay a Day Keep Asthma or Arthritis at Bay? New York Times National,* April 14, 1999, p. A19.

Herbert, Victor (music) and Rida Young (lyrics). *Ah! Sweet Mystery of Life* from *Naughty Marietta.* MGM 1935.

Bibliography

Herzog, RoseAnne. *Unlikely Entrepreneurs: A Business Start-up Guide for People with Disabilities & Chronic Health Conditions.* 1998. North Peak Publishing. pp. 7-32.

Hoffman, Bryce G. *The Detroit News,* May 16, 2006.

Lisle, Douglas J. Ph.D. and Alan Goldhamer, D.C. *The Pleasure Trap: Mastering the Hidden Force that Undermines Health & Happiness.* 2003. Healthy Living Publications, Tennessee.

McCain, John and Marshall Salter. *Why Courage Matters: The Way to a Braver Life.* 2004. Random House, New York. pp. 4-12, 39, 197-199.

Jampolsky, Gerald G. *Love is Letting Go of Fear.* 1981. Bantam Books.

Johnson, Thomas H, ed. 1955. *The Complete Poems of Emily Dickinson,* No. 657, 1862.

Journal of the American Dietary Association, 2003;103: 748-765.

Mindszenty, Jozsef Cardinal. *Memoirs.* English Translation. 1974. Macmillan Publishing.

Myasthenia Gravis Foundation of America, Inc. (800 541-5454) http://www.myasthenia.org

Obese are More than Three Times as Likely to Need a Hip or Knee Replacement, August 17, 2005. Canadian Institute for Health Information.

Page, Vicky. *Learning to Live with Cerebral Palsy,* Story Corps: Recording America, National Public Radio's Morning Edition, May 20, 2005.

Pope John Paul II, *Canonization Mass of Edith Stein,* Vatican City, October 11, 1998, Vatican Information Service.

Red Meat Increases Risk of Rheumatoid Arthritis, Arthritis and Rheumatism, 2004;50:3804-3812.

Thyssen Krupp Budd Co. closes historic east side factory, idles 350 workers. (http://www.detnews.com/apps/pbcs.dll/article?AID=/20060516/AUTO01/605160386/1148)

Warren, Harry and Jack Brooks. *That's Amore.* 1952.

What a Pizza Delivers, Nutrition Action Health Letter of the Center for Science in the Public Interest, June 2002, Vol.29/No.5: 2-9.